BASIC CHILD HEALTH PRACTICE PAPERS
Second edition

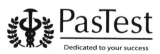

PasTest

Dedicated to your success

BASIC CHILD HEALTH PRACTICE PAPERS
Second Edition

Peter de Halpert MBBS (London) MRCPCH
Specialist Registrar in Paediatrics
North Thames Deanery

Ian Pollock MBBS MRCP FRCPCH DCH DRCOG
Consultant Paediatrician
Barnet and Chase Farm Hospitals NHS Trust

DCH CLINICAL SECTION BY

Austin Isaacs MBBS MSc MRCPCH
Consultant Paediatrician
Barnet and Chase Farm Hospitals NHS Trust

CHILD DEVELOPMENT SECTION BY

Austin Isaacs
and
Rajat Kapoor BMedsci (Hons) BM BS DCH MRCPCH (Part 2)
Senior House Officer in Paediatrics
Barnet and Chase Farm Hospitals NHS Trust

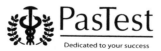

PasTest
Dedicated to your success

© 2007 PasTest Ltd
Egerton Court
Parkgate Estate
Knutsford
Cheshire, WA16 8DX

Telephone: 01565 752000

First edition 2004
Second edition 2007

ISBN: 1 905635 11 7
ISBN: 978 1 905635 11 5

A catalogue record for this book is available from the British Library.

The information contained within this book was obtained by the authors from reliable sources. However, while every effort has been made to ensure its accuracy, no responsibility for loss, damage or injury occasioned to any person acting or refraining from action as a result of information contained herein can be accepted by the publisher or the authors.

PasTest Revision Books and Intensive Courses

PasTest has been established in the field of postgraduate medical education since 1972, providing revision books and intensive study courses for doctors preparing for their professional examinations. Books and courses are available for the following specialties:

MRCP Part 1 and Part 2, MRCPCH Part 1 and Part 2, MRCOG, DRCOG, MRCGP, MRCPsych, DCH, FRCA, MRCS and PLAB.

For further details contact:

PasTest Ltd, Freepost, Knutsford, Cheshire, WA16 7BR
Tel: 01565 752000   Fax: 01565 650264
Email: enquiries@pastest.co.uk   **Web site:** www. pastest.co.uk

Typeset by Breeze Ltd, Manchester
Printed and bound in the UK by Athenaeum Press, Gateshead

CONTENTS

ACKNOWLEDGEMENTS

The second edition of Basic Child Health – Practice Papers is updated to reflect the shift in emphasis by the Royal College of Paediatrics and Child Health towards a higher proportion of 'Best of Five' and Extended Matching Questions. These types of questions are aimed to assess judgement and experience more than pure factual knowledge (best assessed by true/false MCQs). All previous questions have been reviewed and updated to reflect current thinking and clinical practice.

This book is for Sarah and Joe

Peter de Halpert

This book is for Joseph

Ian Pollock

NOTES ON PASSING THE BASIC CHILD HEALTH EXAM

The Diploma of Child Health (DCH) examination is run by the Royal College of Paediatrics and Child Health. It is designed to give recognition of competence in the care of children to general practitioner vocational trainees, staff grades and senior house officers in paediatrics and trainees in specialties allied to paediatrics. The aim is to test knowledge of primary care paediatrics, especially from the following aspects: epidemiology, prenatal care, nutrition and feeding, growth and development, immunisation and screening, health surveillance and promotion, accident prevention, child abuse and legislation, as well as the diagnosis and management of the principal childhood conditions.

THE EXAMINATION

Candidates are advised to have completed a minimum of 6 months' work experience in Paediatrics and Child Health before sitting the examination, because it is unlikely that a candidate would be successful without this experience. The examination consists of two sections:

Written Section – Basic Child Health (Paper 1A):

- 35 True/false Multiple Choice Questions
- 8 Extended Matching Questions
- 25 Best of Five Questions

Paper 1A is taken by candidates for the DCH and the Membership of the Royal College of Paediatrics and Child Health (MRCPCH). Candidates for MRCPCH also have to sit Paper 1B (Extended Paediatrics); these two parts constitute the MRCPCH Part 1.

Candidates who have passed either the MRCP (UK) Part 1 examination or Part 1 of the MRCPCH within the previous 7 years are exempt from the Written section of the DCH examination.

Clinical Section:

From March 2006 the format of the DCH Clinical examination will have changed. There will be eight clinical stations, as follows:

- 2 × Communications, Structured oral, Focused history
- 2 × Short clinical, Neurodevelopment/Neurodisability and Child development

There are 12 objective assessments per candidates and 1 examiner at each station. To pass the examination candidates will need to obtain a total of 118 marks.

Note that, once candidates have passed the MRCPCH Part I Paper 1a, they are then eligible to take the DCH Clinical Examination. Candidates have three attempts at the DCH Clinical Examination. Once all three attempts have been exhausted candidates must re-sit MRCPCH Part I Paper 1a.

THE WRITTEN PAPERS

Multiple Choice Questions

There are 35 questions, each having five stems that are either 'True' or 'False'. One mark (+) is awarded for each correct answer, and so a total of five marks is possible for each question. There is NO negative marking, so if you do not know the answer it is always worth putting an answer down, because a 'don't know' or no answer at all will not get you any marks. Remember to read each stem carefully and look out for terms such as 'always/never' (generally False) and 'may/can' (generally True). Usually a brief outline is provided of a common condition found in primary care, followed by four or five questions, often interjected with new information as the story unfolds. However, always answer the question at the stage that it is posed without the influence of forthcoming information. Although knowledge of medical management is important, the focus is more on the psychosocial aspects of care of the child and his or her family. It is essential to be familiar with the roles of each member of the multidisciplinary team and to be able to advise on health education and prevention, etc.

Extended Matching Questions

Ten possible answers are listed followed by three scenarios. A question asks for the most correct answer from the list (much the same way as the Best of Five – see below). Each of these questions is worth 9 marks (3 per item).

It is worth noting that, as these questions test judgement/experience, some clinicians may not necessarily agree with some of the answers given in this book. This is not to say that the answers here are flawed, just that the answers given are correct in our opinion. Candidates are advised that these practice papers should not form the basis of a revision programme – but should be used as a guide to what the actual questions may be like.

It is worth noting that to provide a list of 10 possible answers, sometimes some of the answers listed may be slightly esoteric/uncommon. This paper is designed to test what a candidate is likely to have seen in 6–12 months of hospital, community or primary care paediatrics. If a rare or uncommon cause is listed, it may well be a possible answer but it is worth considering that it may be less likely because the paper is not designed to test extended paediatrics.

Best of Five Questions

These questions are designed to test experience and judgement. A short statement is followed by five possible answers, all of which could be right. The candidate must choose the answer that is the most right. Each of these questions is worth 4 marks.

Again these questions represent our own opinions.

PAPER I

MULTIPLE CHOICE QUESTIONS

1.1 With regard to congenital hypertrophic pyloric stenosis:

○ A It has an incidence of 4 per 1000 live births
○ B It typically presents with projectile bile-stained vomiting
○ C It is more common in girls
○ D It may cause hyperkalaemic alkalosis
○ E The investigation of choice is ultrasonography

1.2 In children the features of nephrotic syndrome include:

○ A Proteinuria, hypoalbuminaemia, generalised oedema and hyperlipidaemia
○ B The most common cause of idiopathic (primary) nephrotic syndrome being diffuse proliferative glomerulonephritis
○ C Serum albumin < 35 g/L
○ D Strict adherence to a high-protein, no-salt diet is needed
○ E A peak incidence at between 2 and 5 years of age

1.3 With regard to low-birthweight (LBW) infants:

○ A Premature infants are those born before 36 completed weeks' gestation
○ B Very-low-birthweight infants are those weighing < 2500 g
○ C There is a characteristic association with maternal diabetes
○ D They have an increased incidence of congenital malformations
○ E Babies who are small for gestational age (SGA) may reflect maternal diabetes

1

1.4   With regard to tonsils and adenoids:

○   A   Purulent follicular exudate is present only in bacterial
            tonsillitis

○   B   A 3-day course of penicillin is adequate treatment for
            bacterial tonsillitis

○   C   Recurrent febrile convulsions associated with attacks of
            follicular tonsillitis are an indication for a tonsillectomy

○   D   Primary post-tonsillectomy haemorrhage is usually the
            result of infection

○   E   Adenoidectomy is useful in the treatment of glue ear

1.5   With regard to autism:

○   A   Males and females are equally affected

○   B   It usually develops after 3 years of age

○   C   Drugs such as tranquillisers have a common role in the
            management of children with autism

○   D   Autistic children commonly have islands of intact
            intellectual functioning – the so-called idiot savant

○   E   A diagnosis of autism can be made if the child has two of
            the following features:
            – global impairment of language and communication
            – impairment of social relationships, especially empathy
            – ritualistic and compulsive phenomena

**1.6   In an 8-year-old girl presenting with staining of her
        underwear and slight yellow discharge at the introitus
        with no other signs:**

○   A   It is urgent to exclude sexual abuse in the first instance

○   B   Vulvovaginitis is the most likely diagnosis

○   C   *Gardnerella vaginalis* is a common infecting organism

○   D   Lack of labial fat pads protecting the vaginal orifice and
            the excess acidity of the prepubertal vagina are increased
            risk factors for infection

○   E Topical dienestrol cream is a useful treatment

1.7   **With regard to blood pressure measurement in children:**

○   A It should be a routine part of a cardiovascular examination

○   B The correct cuff size is approximately two-thirds the length of the upper arm

○   C The fifth Korotkoff sound is used for diastolic measurement

○   D Raised blood pressure in children aged < 6 years is commonly the result of primary hypertension

○   E A diastolic pressure > 90 mmHg before age 13 years requires treatment

1.8   **With regard to cot death/near miss cot death:**

○   A If an infant suffers a cot death but the twin appears in excellent health, the parents may be reassured

○   B Apnoea monitors do not decrease the incidence of cot death

○   C Risk factors include viral infections, prone sleeping position, hypothermia and old polyvinyl chloride (PVC) mattresses

○   D Parents should be taught to recognise and assess signs of illness in their babies and be discouraged from frequent visits to the general practitioner (GP) that may result in increased anxiety

○   E Parents who stop smoking significantly decrease the risk of their child suffering a cot death

questions

1.9   With regard to acute bronchiolitis:

○ A Up to 50% of cases are caused by the respiratory syncytial virus (RSV)

○ B Nasopharyngeal aspirate may be used for the direct detection of virus in secretions by immunofluorescence

○ C Ribavirin is an antiviral agent effective against RSV and should be used as a first-line treatment if RSV infection is confirmed

○ D Salbutamol and theophylline have no effect on bronchiolar obstruction under 1 year of age

○ E Maternal immunoglobulin IgA is protective against RSV

1.10   With regard to eczema:

○ A In 70% there is a family history of atopy

○ B It resolves by 5 years in 80% of children

○ C It often starts on the face/neck/behind the ears, but favours extensor surfaces in older children

○ D Chinese herbal therapy is of proven benefit in resistant cases

○ E Breast-feeding or hypoallergenic formula milk decreases the risk and severity in infants with a positive family history of atopy

1.11   With regard to school refusal:

○ A It is most common in children aged 11–14 years

○ B Children typically come from social classes I and II

○ C It is more common in girls

○ D It commonly presents with recurrent abdominal pains or headaches

○ E It typically occurs in a conscientious and intelligent student

1.12 Causes of persistent snoring in children include:

○   A Hypertrophic nasal turbinates
○   B Hyperthyroidism
○   C Obesity
○   D Down's syndrome
○   E Recurrent tonsillitis

1.13 With regard to oesophageal atresia (OA):

○   A Of affected babies 85% will have a tracheo-oesophageal
         fistula
○   B It may be associated with cardiovascular and urogenital
         anomalies
○   C Mothers often have oligohydramnios antenatally
○   D It can present with recurrent pneumonia
○   E It is diagnosed by a barium swallow

1.14 With regard to reflexes:

○   A The Moro reflex persists from birth to about 3 months
○   B The rooting/suckling and swallowing reflex is usually
         absent before 34/40
○   C An absent red reflex may indicate a retinoblastoma
○   D The grasping reflex persists from birth to about 3 months
○   E The stepping reflex persists from birth to about 6 months

1.15 Treatment of cystic fibrosis includes:

○   A Regular physiotherapy
○   B Heart and lung transplantation
○   C Long-term prophylactic amoxicillin
○   D High-protein, low-fat diet
○   E Pancreatic enzyme supplements with main meals only

1.16 With regard to screening criteria:

A   A screening test should have low sensitivity and specificity

B   Acceptable screening tests should give a yield of at least 1 in 100 000

C   Screening tests should be inexpensive

D   Effective screening tests are available for most conditions

E   Screening must be a continuous process

1.17 Features of a headache that would alert you to the diagnosis of serious intracranial pathology are:

A   Transient ataxia, hemiparesis or aphasia

B   Recent onset of a squint

C   If it wakes the child at night and is most severe first thing in the morning

D   Relief on implementing an 'exclusion diet' (ie chocolate, cheese, milk, etc)

E   Deterioration in school performance

1.18 Causes of short stature include:

A   Noonan syndrome

B   Soto syndrome

C   Turner's syndrome

D   Klinefelter syndrome

E   Marfan syndrome

1.19 Conditions that may result in a false-positive sweat test include:

A   Addison's disease

B   Hypothyroidism

C   Diabetes mellitus

D   Nephrogenic diabetes insipidus

E   Bronchiectasis

1.20 The Education Act 1993:

○   A   Defines a child with special educational needs (SENs) as one who has a learning difficulty that requires special educational provision to be made

○   B   States that children whose language of the home is different from the one in which they will be taught may be considered to have a learning difficulty

○   C   States that children with SENs should be taught in special schools

○   D   Requires a statement of SENs to be made and reviewed regularly

○   E   States that special educational provision includes any educational provision given to a child aged under 2 years

1.21 Concerning accidents:

○   A   They are the single largest cause of death in children aged between 1 and 14 years

○   B   Of all childhood deaths 60% are the result of accidents

○   C   The most common fatal accidents are caused by falls

○   D   About 15% of all children a year attend A&E because of an accidental injury

○   E   The incidence is similar in boys and girls

1.22 With regard to bilirubin toxicity:

○   A   It is caused by free unconjugated bilirubin, which is lipid soluble and therefore readily diffuses across brain cell membranes

○   B   Kernicterus occurs only when the serum bilirubin exceeds 380 mmol/L

○   C   The symptoms include hypotonia and lethargy

○   D   If the baby survives, long-term sequelae include choreo-athetoid cerebral palsy and high-frequency nerve deafness

○   E   Phototherapy uses a narrow-spectrum blue light of wavelength 450–475 nm

questions

1.23 The following drugs are safe in breast-feeding:

- A Thyroxine
- B Digoxin
- C Nitrazepam
- D Cimetidine
- E Chlorpheniramine

1.24 Recognised causes of epistaxis in children include:

- A Nose picking
- B Hypertension
- C Upper respiratory tract infection
- D Allergic rhinitis
- E Foreign bodies

1.25 Concerning dentition:

- A There are 32 deciduous teeth
- B Teething causes fever, irritability and excessive salivation
- C Children do not have the hand–eye coordination to clean their teeth adequately until about 8–10 years of age
- D The first tooth to appear is generally a lower central incisor
- E Malocclusion may result from thumb sucking

1.26 With regard to urinary tract infections (UTIs):

- A They may present with vomiting, irritability and feeding problems
- B They should be investigated during or after a child's second UTI
- C Urine specimens can be stored at 0–4°C for up to 24 h
- D The presence of pyuria proves a UTI
- E Obesity predisposes to UTI in girls

1.27 With regard to scabies:

- A It is caused by the *Sarcoptes scabiei* mite
- B Burrows usually involve the interdigital webs or flexor aspects of the wrists, while sparing the face and scalp of infants
- C Only symptomatic family members need to be treated
- D Itching is usually worse at night
- E Persistent pruritus 2 weeks later implies failure of treatment

1.28 With regard to obesity:

- A It is associated with growth hormone deficiency
- B It may be complicated by Blount's disease
- C It is associated with Lawrence–Moon–Biedl syndrome
- D Most obese healthy children are tall for their age
- E It is associated with hyperparathyroidism

1.29 Management of epilepsy includes:

- A Ketogenic diet
- B Discouraging swimming
- C Wearing protective helmets while cycling alone on open roads
- D Surgery
- E Education in normal schools

1.30 Causes of constipation include:

- A Congenital absence of intestinal autonomic ganglion cells of the Auerbach and Messnier plexus
- B Dehydration
- C Hypocalcaemia
- D Hypothyroidism
- E Over-enthusiastic potty training

questions

1.31 Phenylketonuria:

- A Is an autosomal dominant condition
- B Is associated with infantile spasms
- C Is detected using the Guthrie test at approximately day 6
- D Will result in mental disability if the diagnosis is delayed
- E May harm normal infants *in utero* if their affected mothers do not maintain their dietary restrictions throughout the pregnancy

1.32 The following are notifiable diseases:

- A Acquired immune deficiency syndrome (AIDS)
- B Mumps
- C Tuberculosis (TB)
- D Rubella
- E Malaria

1.33 With regard to acute lymphoblastic leukaemia (ALL):

- A It accounts for 85% of all childhood leukaemias
- B It commonly presents with bone and joint pain
- C It is more common in girls
- D The presence of a B-cell immunological surface membrane marker is associated with the best prognosis
- E Epstein–Barr virus is associated with an increased risk of developing leukaemia

1.34 With regard to spina bifida:

○   A   Spina bifida occulta is seen in 5–10% of all children's spines

○   B   Arnold–Chiari malformation is frequently associated with myelomeningocele

○   C   Myelomeningocele characteristically causes spastic paraplegia of the lower limbs

○   D   Meningocele has no neurological involvement

○   E   Myelomeningocele is characteristically associated with incontinence of urine, but not of faeces

1.35 Which of the following incubation periods are correct?

○   A   Chickenpox: 2–5 days

○   B   Measles: 7–14 days

○   C   Glandular fever: 14–21 days

○   D   Mumps: 12–31 days

○   E   Rubella: 7–14 days

questions

EXTENDED MATCHING QUESTIONS

1.36 Theme: analysis of blood gases

○ A Compensated metabolic acidosis
○ B Compensated respiratory acidosis
○ C Metabolic acidosis
○ D Metabolic alkalosis
○ E Mixed metabolic/respiratory acidosis
○ F Mixed metabolic/respiratory alkalosis
○ G Partially compensated metabolic acidosis
○ H Partially compensated respiratory acidosis
○ I Respiratory acidosis
○ J Respiratory alkalosis

For each of the following cases, please choose the most appropriate analysis of the blood gas results from the above list (each item may be used once or not at all):

1   An ex-23-weeks' gestation baby is discharged with home oxygen. His venous blood gas analysis before discharge shows: pH 7.39, $Paco_2$ 12.1 kPa, Pao_2 6.1 kPa, HCO_3^- 42 mmol/L, BE (base excess) +13 mmol/L.

2   A 6-year-old child with known diabetes presents with an intercurrent illness. His BM (blood glucose testing strip) is 25 and an arterial blood gas shows: pH 7.32, $Paco_2$ 2.9 kPa, Pao_2 10.2 kPa, Hco_3^- 18 mmol/L, BE -7 mmol/L.

3   A 7-week-old newborn girl presents with vomiting. A capillary blood gas shows pH 7.46, $Paco_2$ 6.4 kPa, Pao_2 5.5 kPa, Hco_3^- 38 mmol/L, BE +4 mmol/L.

1.37 Theme: immunisation

○ A No live vaccines
○ B No vaccines at all
○ C Normal immunisation schedule D
○ D Normal schedule with separate pertussis vaccine
○ E Normal schedule without BCG (Bacille Camille–Guérin)
○ F Normal schedule and unconjugated pneumococcal immunisation
○ G Normal schedule without polio vaccine
○ H Normal schedule with substitution of single vaccines for MMR (measles, mumps, rubella)
○ I Normal schedule without MMR
○ J Normal schedule without MMR or BCG

For each of the following children, please choose the most appropriate immunisation policy from the above list (each item may be used more than once):

1 A child born in the UK with vertically acquired human immunodeficiency virus (HIV) infection.
2 A child diagnosed on the autistic spectrum.
3 A child who has sickle cell trait.

1.38 Theme: infant milk formulae

- ◯ A Breast milk
- ◯ B Elemental formula
- ◯ C 'Follow-on' milk
- ◯ D Goats' milk
- ◯ E High-energy formula
- ◯ F Hydrolysed protein formula
- ◯ G Pre-term infant formula
- ◯ H Term infant formula
- ◯ I Soya infant formula
- ◯ J Soya milk

For each of the following cases, please choose the most appropriate milk from the above list (each item may be used once or not at all):

1   A 7-month-old infant who has chronic lung disease of prematurity and is on home O_2 and is failing to thrive on term infant formula.

2   A newborn baby whose mother has hepatitis C.

3   A 2-month-old baby who suffers from gastro-oesophageal reflux, is failing to thrive and has a sibling who 'can't have dairy'.

1.39 Theme: epilepsy

○ A Absence epilepsy
○ B Complex partial seizures (of the temporal lobe)
○ C Febrile convulsion
○ D Idiopathic generalised tonic–clonic epilepsy
○ E Infantile spasms
○ F Night terror
○ G Partial seizure
○ H Pseudoseizure
○ I Rigors
○ J Rolandic epilepsy

For each of the following cases, please choose the most likely diagnosis from the above list (each item may be used once or not at all):

1 A 8-year-old boy develops generalised tonic–clonic seizures. They occur any time during the day and can occur at night. He has centrotemporal spikes on EEG.

2 The EEG of 5-year-old child with poor concentration at school shows a 3/s spike-and-wave discharge provoked by hyperventilation.

3 A 6-year-old child has episodes of nausea and abdominal pain, followed by repetitive chewing and jerking of the left arm for 1–2 min. He is confused afterwards.

1.40 Theme: rashes

○ A Erysipelas
○ B Hand, foot and mouth disease
○ C Infectious mononucleosis
○ D Measles
○ E Molluscum contagiosum
○ F Pityriasis rosea
○ G Rubella
○ H Sixth disease
○ I Slapped cheek syndrome
○ J Varicella-zoster

For each of the following clinical scenarios, please choose the most likely diagnosis from the above list (each item may be used once or not at all):

1   A 5-year-old boy presents with a macular rash on the trunk; some of the macules run parallel to his ribs. His mother reports that 5 days ago there was only one spot that must have spread.

2   A 4-year-old child is systemically unwell; she has erythematous cheeks that are hot and very tender to touch.

3   A 14-month-old baby girl presents with a fine pink macular rash that started on her face and spread to her trunk. Cervical and occipital lymph nodes are easily palpable.

17

questions

1.41 Theme: renal diseases

- ○ A Bartter syndrome
- ○ B Factitious illness
- ○ C Haemolytic uraemic syndrome (HUS)
- ○ D Henoch–Schönlein purpura (HSP) nephritis
- ○ E Mesangial IgA nephropathy
- ○ F Nephrotic syndrome
- ○ G Post-streptococcal glomerulonephritis
- ○ H Reflux nephropathy
- ○ I Systemic lupus erythematosus (SLE)
- ○ J UTI

For each of the following clinical scenarios, please choose the most likely diagnosis from the above list (each item may be used once or not at all):

1 A 4-year-old child is brought to see you as his mother noticed that his urine is pink. He has been complaining of headaches. His blood pressure is 130/88 mmHg. Blood tests reveal: Na^+ 130 mmol/L, K^+ 4.9 mmol/L, urea (Ur) 12 mmol/L, creatinine (Cr) 96 µmol/L. Complement C3 is reduced but C4 is normal. Albumin is 29 g/L.

2 A 13-year-old child presents with blood in the urine. He reports having an upper respiratory tract infection (URTI) 3 days ago. His blood pressure is 120/60 mmHg. Urine analysis reveals only blood 3+, protein 2+. Renal function is normal. Complement levels are normal.

3 A 6-year-old child who has had diarrhoea for the past week is brought to A&E. Her baseline bloods reveal: Na^+ 133 mmol/L, K^+ 5.4 mmol/L, Cr 90 µmol/L, Ur 42 mmol/L, Hb 6.3 g/dL, white cell count (WCC) 2.3×10^9/L, platelets (plts) 95×10^9/L.

1.42 Theme: the unwell infant

- ○ A Cardiac failure
- ○ B Congenital toxoplasmosis
- ○ C Delayed group B streptococcal sepsis
- ○ D Delayed haemorrhagic disease of the newborn
- ○ E Duct-dependent cardiac lesion
- ○ F Galactosaemia
- ○ G Hereditary lactic acidosis
- ○ H Meningitis
- ○ I Non-accidental injury (NAI)
- ○ J Wilson's disease

For each of the following 'unwell infant' scenarios, please choose the most likely diagnosis from the above list (each item may be used once or not at all):

1   A 3-week-old baby is brought to A&E; he has recently been having problems completing his feeds and today appears short of breath. On examination he has 4-cm hepatomegaly. All blood tests are normal.

2   A 2-week-old baby boy presents to A&E; he looks unwell. He is jaundiced, peripherally shut down and has hepatosplenomegaly. Baseline investigations show: Hb 8 g/dL, WCC 2.9 × 10^9/L, plts 120 × 10^9/L, international normalised ratio (INR) 8.6, γ-glutamyl transferase (γ-GT) 300 IU/L, BM 2.3, urine reducing sugars +ve.

3   A 6-week-old bottle-fed baby boy attends A&E with his parents. His father reports that he is always crying. On examination he is afebrile, irritable and has a bulging fontanelle. Urgent computed tomography (CT) (brain) shows multiple haemorrhages and generalised oedema.

1.43 Theme: immunodeficiency

○ A IgA deficiency
○ B Severe combined immunodeficiency
○ C Selective IgG deficiency
○ D Chronic granulomatous disease
○ E HIV infection
○ F Bruton's agammaglobinaemia
○ G DiGeorge syndrome
○ H Wiskott–Aldrich syndrome
○ I Ataxia telangiectasia
○ J Leukocyte adhesion defect

From the list above, select the most likely diagnosis for each of the cases below:

1   A 3-year-old is seen in clinic after two previous admissions for pneumonia. He recently had grommets inserted. His parents report that he always has a runny nose. You know that he has eczema but no other skin lesions.

2   A 3-and-a-half-year old boy is admitted for atypical pneumonia. His mother says that he has recurrent diarrhoea. On examination you note that he is growth faltering and that he also has severe oral candidiasis.

3   A 4-month-old African child presents with growth faltering. On examination he is noted to have eczema and oral candidiasis. The full blood count (FBC) is normal. IgG is raised, IgM low and IgA low.

BEST OF FIVE QUESTIONS

1.44 A newborn infant is noted to be profoundly hypotonic at birth; he has a good heart rate but is in respiratory distress. Which of the following syndromes is most likely to be the cause?

○ A Down's syndrome
○ B Prader–Willi syndrome
○ C Noonan syndrome
○ D Werdnig–Hoffman disease (spinomuscular atrophy type 1)
○ E Beckwith–Wiedemann syndrome

1.45 In a child whose asthma is not controlled on a regular inhaled steroid and occasional β2 agonist, the single next best step would be to:

○ A Add a long-acting β2 agonist
○ B Increase the dose of inhaled steroid
○ C Check the inhaler technique
○ D Add a leukotriene inhibitor
○ E Add a short course of oral steroids

1.46 A 4-month-old infant presents with a fever, cough and reduced feeds. Her respiratory rate is 60/min with mild recession, wheeze and crackles throughout. The most likely diagnosis is:

○ A Croup
○ B Virally induced atopic wheeze
○ C Cystic fibrosis
○ D Bacterial chest infection
○ E Bronchiolitis

questions

questions

1.47 **Which of the following statements is most correct with regard to the consent for an operation on a 10-year-old child whose parents aren't married?**

○ A Either of the parents or the child can consent to the operation

○ B Either of the parents but not the child can consent to the operation

○ C Only the mother or the child can consent to the operation

○ D Only the mother can consent to the operation

○ E Only the child can consent to the operation

1.48 **Which of the following is the first sign of puberty in girls?**

○ A Menarche

○ B Breast development

○ C Growth spurt

○ D Axillary hair development

○ E Pubic hair development

1.49 **A 7-year-old boy presents with pain in his right leg. He is afebrile. On examination you note that the range of movement in his right hip is limited by pain. The most likely diagnosis is:**

○ A Perthes' disease

○ B Irritable hip

○ C Septic arthritis

○ D Slipped upper femoral epiphysis (SUFE)

○ E Osgood–Schlatter disease

1.50 **Which of the following statements best describes clinical governance?**

○   A   Performance of audit, audit direct process change and completion of cycles

○   B   Comprehensive risk assessment and incident reporting

○   C   Implementation and systematic review of clinical effectiveness

○   D   Modification of healthcare systems to optimise patient care

○   E   Systematic training of healthcare workers to effect quality provision

1.51 **A child with congenital hypothyroidism is currently on 50 µg/day thyroxine (T4). She is seen in clinic and has the following thyroid function tests (TFTs): free T_4 20.2 (12–24) nmol/L, thyroid-stimulating hormone (TSH) 9.8 (1.2–4.0) mU/L. Which of the following explanations is the most likely?**

○   A   Under-treatment

○   B   Over-treatment

○   C   Anti-T_4 antibodies

○   D   Poor compliance

○   E   Wrong diagnosis

questions

1.52 A parent suspects that her 2-year-old son has a food intolerance and wants 'tests'. He is well and growing along the appropriate centile. What is the most appropriate course of action?

A Advise her that there are no investigations that can 100% determine food intolerances

B Advise her to try to exclude the suspected food and see if this produces an improvement in his symptoms; if so then reintroduce and see if the symptoms return

C Perform skin-prick testing to the suspected allergen and other common allergens

D Perform radioallergosorbent test (RAST) to the suspected allergens and other common allergens

E Perform baseline coeliac screen, stool-reducing sugars and inflammatory markers to exclude more serious pathology

1.53 A 2-month-old baby girl is brought to your surgery because her mother is concerned about a 1 cm lump situated lateral to her right eyebrow. The lump is firm and not attached to the skin. Which of the following lumps is the most likely diagnosis?

A Enlarged lymph node
B Lipoma
C Branchial cyst
D External angular dermoid
E Neurofibroma

1.54 Which of the following gross motor milestones would you expect a normally developing 10-month-old infant to have most recently acquired?

A Sitting unsupported
B Pulling to stand
C Rolling prone to supine
D Walking up stairs with support

○ E Transferring hand to hand

1.55 Which of the following fine motor milestones would you expect a normally developing 20-month-old infant to have most recently acquired?

○ A Casting
○ B Thumb/finger grip
○ C Banging two cubes together
○ D Feeding self with a spoon
○ E Building a tower of two cubes

1.56 A 3-year-old girl was hit by a reversing car (5 mph). She sustained a head injury and loss of consciousness for 1 min. Subsequent to this she has vomited three times. On examination, her Glasgow Coma Scale (GCS) score is 15/15 and there is no focal neurology. Which of the following is the most appropriate course of action?

○ A Discharge with head injury advice for the parents
○ B Arrange urgent computed tomography (CT) of her brain
○ C Arrange anteroposterior (AP) and lateral skull radiographs
○ D Admit for 24 hours of neurological observations
○ E Observe for 4 hours in A&E and then send home with head injury advice if well

1.57 Which of the following language milestones would you expect 90% of normally developing children to have most recently developed by 1 year?

○ A Turning to voice
○ B Imitating speech sounds
○ C Three words
○ D Dada/mama (specific to person)
○ E Expressive babbling

1.58 Which of the following tests is the most appropriate to check the hearing of a 5-year-old child?

- A Auditory brain-stem-evoked response
- B Distraction test
- C Otoacoustic emissions
- D Pure-tone audiometry
- E Impedance audiometry

1.59 A 3-month-old baby girl is brought to your clinic because her mother is concerned that her birthmark is still present. On examination she has a capillary haemangioma on her left thigh. Which of the following statements is the most appropriate to tell the mother?

- A The birthmark should resolve by 5 years of age
- B The birthmark may get larger until 2 years of age then resolve by 5 years
- C The birthmark may get larger until 2 years of age then resolve by 10 years
- D The birthmark may get larger until 2 years of age and probably will have gone by 5 years but may never resolve completely
- E The birthmark may get larger until 2 years of age, and 70% resolve by 5 years and 95% by 10 years

1.60 Which of the following investigations is the one that has the greatest relevance to the ophthalmic monitoring of a child with juvenile idiopathic arthritis?

- A Anti-neutrophil cytoplasmic antibodies (ANCAs)
- B Erythrocyte sedimentation rate (ESR)
- C C-reactive protein (CRP)
- D Anti-nuclear antibodies (ANAs)
- E Extractable nuclear antigens

1.61 Which of the following is, ideally, the most appropriate insulin regimen for a 3-year-old child newly diagnosed as having type 1 diabetes?

A Basal–bolus regimen

B Twice daily (30% short/70% intermediate acting): at $2/_3$ of dose am and $1/_3$ of dose pm

C Twice daily (20% short/80% intermediate acting): at $1/_2$ of dose am and $1/_2$ of dose pm

D Once-daily long-acting insulin

E Three times daily, short-acting insulin

1.62 A 7-month-old baby boy from the Indian subcontinent has been in the UK for 1 month. At a routine health visit he is noted to be pale. Subsequent investigations show FBC: Hb 9.3 g/dL, WCC 4.5 × 10^9/L, plts 240 × 10^9/L, mean corpuscular volume (MCV) 70 fL, ferritin 16 ng/mL (normal range 100–500 ng/mL), reticulocytes 1.6%, Hb electrophoresis 98% HbA. Given these results, what is the most likely cause for the anaemia?

A Physiological anaemia of infancy

B α-Thalassaemia trait

C Chronic helminthic infection

D Dietary iron deficiency

E Dietary folate deficiency

questions

1.63 A 4-year-old child presents after a viral URTI with bruising and petechiae, but is afebrile and well. On examination there are petechiae on the trunk and legs, bruises on the leg, no petechiae in the mouth or lips, and no other abnormal findings. His platelet count is 9×10^9/L; the rest of the FBC, coagulation screen and urine dipstick are normal. A diagnosis of ITP (immune-mediated thrombocytopenic purpura) is made. What is the best course of action from this point?

A Admit and observe for 48 h with daily platelet counts

B Admit and start intravenous immunoglobulin

C Admit and start intravenous immunoglobulin followed by 1 unit platelets

D Admit and arrange for a bone marrow aspiration, with a view to starting steroids

E Discharge home but arrange for daily review and FBC

1.64 A mother brings her 4-and-a-half-month-old boy to your clinic. She complains that for the last week he has been 'grizzly all the time', 'putting his thumbs and fingers in his mouth and will chew anything he's given'. He was previously sleeping for 7 h at night but now wakes twice for feeds. She has been applying a topical anti-inflammatory to his gums. On examination there is no specific finding of note; the infant is afebrile and generally robust. What is the most appropriate advice to give?

A This is teething – there is no specific treatment

B This is likely to be a viral URTI

C This is a normal occurrence at this age, and in the absence of any abnormal findings reassurance should be given

D The infant is clearly underfed and should be weaned

E The infant needs to be referred for developmental assessment

1.65 A 5-year-old girl has had a persistent nocturnal cough for over 2 years, which has not responded to treatment including inhaled steroids and bronchodilators. The cough tends to be paroxysmal and is associated with vomiting, disturbing her sleep virtually every night. She is happy and normally active during the day and does not have any exercise intolerance. In other respects she has been well with no significant past history. There is no family history of asthma, eczema or allergy. Her weight is on the 75th centile and height on the 50th centile. General and systematic examinations are normal. Chest radiograph is essentially normal. FBC within the normal range, ESR 12 mm, CRP 5 mg, peak expiratory flow (PEF) 90% predicted, Mantoux negative. The next most useful investigation that will aid the diagnosis is:

A   Bronchoscopy
B   Spirometry
C   Barium meal
D   Ambulatory oesophageal pH study
E   CT of thorax

1.66 You are called about a day-old baby on the postnatal ward; he is yet to have a baby check. The mother has revealed recreational drug use in her pregnancy. She is happy for urine toxicology to be sent on the baby. The baby's father arrives and is angry at this, and is threatening to take the mother and baby home against medical advice. The parents are unmarried. What is the best course of action?

A   Call security to stop them leaving so you can assess the baby
B   Call the police to stop them leaving so you can assess the baby
C   Allow them to leave but ask the GP to check on the baby
D   Allow them to leave but inform the duty social worker
E   Allow them to leave and take no further action

questions

1.67 An 18-month-old boy presents with poor feeding and tachypnoea a week after a coryzal illness. His cardiac examination is unremarkable, other than a third heart sound being present. His chest radiograph shows cardiomegaly and bilateral interstitial shadowing. FBC, renal function and anti-streptolysin O test (ASOT) are normal. What is the most likely diagnosis?

A Coxsackie myocarditis

B Lyme disease

C Parvovirus B19 infection

D Rheumatic fever

E Kawasaki's disease

1.68 A set of twins are brought to see you aged 5 days. They are being exclusively breast-fed. They are both jaundiced, requiring admission for phototherapy, and have lost 12% and 13% of their birthweights, respectively. They both have serum sodium levels of 145 mmol/L. What is the best advice about fluid management over the next 48 h?

A Intravenous 10% dextrose at 150 mL/kg per day

B Continue breast-feeding both of them exclusively

C Continue breast-feeding but give full top-ups via nasogastric tube

D Give them full requirements by bottle or EBM (expressed breast milk) and additional formula if necessary

E Start formula 150 mL/kg per day by bottle

PAPER 2

MULTIPLE CHOICE QUESTIONS

2.1   With regard to consent:

A A child aged less than 16 years may give consent for elective medical treatment

B If a child aged less than 16 years refuses surgery it must not be carried out

C An unmarried father has both financial and intrinsic rights for his child

D If a divorced couple disagree about the need for an elective tonsillectomy in their child, the mother's opinion prevails

E If emergency surgery is needed and the parents are unavailable, consent must be obtained from a person such as a teacher who is *in loco parentis*

2.2   With regard to acne:

A It affects 90% of teenagers and 25% of infants

B It is usually caused by excessive levels of testosterone

C *Propionibacterium acnes* is an anaerobic diphtheroid

D In moderate cases, treatment with erythromycin should continue for at least 6–12 months

E Roaccutane (isotretinoin – a vitamin A analogue) can be tried by the GP for severe cases resistant to all other therapy

questions

2.3 Signs of physical abuse include:

- A Petechial rash over the child's face
- B Torn frenulum
- C Mongolian blue spot
- D Multiple bruising of various ages on the shins of a 7-year-old boy
- E Metaphyseal avulsion fractures

2.4 With regard to Turner's syndrome:

- A It affects 1 in 2500 women
- B It has the genotype XY; however, intrauterine development persists because essentially female as a result of lack of receptors for circulating testosterone
- C It is associated with Crohn's disease
- D Features apparent at birth include a webbed neck, low posterior hairline and widely spaced nipples
- E Somatotrophin (human growth hormone) is a useful treatment for short stature once the epiphyses have fused

2.5 With regard to molluscum contagiosum:

- A It is a pox RNA virus infection
- B It typically presents with small, pearly, umbilicated lesions anywhere on the body
- C It has low infectivity
- D Lesions generally take 6–9 months to resolve
- E The treatment of choice is removal by piercing the lesion with a sharpened orange stick dipped in phenol or liquid nitrogen

questions

2.6 With regard to nappy rash:

○ A It typically involves the flexures when a result of irritant dermatitis

○ B A red rash with satellite lesions and shallow ulcers is typical of candidiasis

○ C It frequently becomes secondarily infected with *Staphylococcus aureus*

○ D Topical Dermovate cream (clobetasol propionate) is the treatment of choice for the scaly intertriginous nappy rash

○ E Nappy rash caused by seborrhoeic dermatitis may be associated with cradle cap

2.7 With regard to factitious or induced illness:

○ A It has a mortality rate of 2–10%
○ B Confrontation with evidence should be avoided
○ C It never involves the father
○ D The child may show evidence of failure to thrive
○ E Generally occurs in pre-school children

2.8 With regard to clubfoot:

○ A It is more common in boys
○ B The feet are held in equinovalgus
○ C It may be associated with spina bifida
○ D It will need surgical repair
○ E Treatment should be commenced at the age of 3 months

2.9 With regard to cleft lip:

○ A It has an equal incidence among boys and girls
○ B It is increasing in incidence
○ C It affects approximately 1 in 750 live births
○ D It is associated with cleft palate in less than 20% of patients
○ E The risk to a child whose sibling has a cleft lip is 5%

2.10 With regard to tonsillectomy:

A It is indicated in children who have two attacks of tonsillitis a year

B Complications include development of a quinsy

C It should be performed if parents request a prophylactic procedure

D Complications include complete dysphagia

E Postoperative secondary haemorrhage is treated with antibiotics

2.11 With regard to Wilms' nephroblastoma:

A It commonly presents before 5 years of age

B It is frequently bilateral

C It often presents with haematuria

D Diagnosis should be confirmed by renal biopsy

E It is the most common intra-abdominal tumour of childhood

2.12 With regard to undescended testis:

A It is present in 15–30% of term male infants

B When present it is usually bilateral

C It is most commonly found at the superficial inguinal pouch

D Orchidopexy should be performed before 4 years of age

E There is an increased incidence of torsion

2.13 Known side effects of sodium valproate include:

A Pancreatitis

B Stevens–Johnson syndrome

C Hyperactivity, commonly

D Increased appetite and obesity

E Epigastric pain and nausea

2.14 An acute asthma attack may be triggered by:

- ○ A Exercise
- ○ B Gastro-oesophageal reflux
- ○ C Climatic change
- ○ D Rhinovirus infection
- ○ E Emotion

2.15 With regard to Bacillus Calmette–Guérin (BCG):

- ○ A High-risk infants should have a positive Heaf test before immunisation proceeds
- ○ B It is safe in asymptomatic HIV-positive patients
- ○ C It may be given at the same time as other live vaccines
- ○ D It should be given after a positive tuberculin test
- ○ E Offers some protection against leprosy

2.16 Congenital rubella is characteristically associated with:

- ○ A Deafness with maternal infection at 10–16 weeks' gestation
- ○ B Retinopathy
- ○ C Hydrocephalus
- ○ D Polycythaemia
- ○ E Neonatal conjugated hyperbilirubinaemia

2.17 Which of these definitions is correct?

- ○ A The 'incidence' of influenza is much lower than its 'prevalence'
- ○ B The 'perinatal mortality' is the number of stillbirths and deaths within the first week of life per 1000 total births
- ○ C 'Stillbirth rate' is the number of stillbirths per 1000 total births
- ○ D 'Neonatal mortality rate' (NMR) is the number of deaths in babies up to 1 month of age per 1000 total births
- ○ E 'Infant mortality rate' (IMR) is the number of deaths in babies under 1 year

questions

2.18 With regard to Apgar scores:

- A   A heart rate of < 100 beats/min scores 1
- B   Approximately 45% of all babies whose Apgar score is < 4 at 5 min will die
- C   They are recorded at 0, 1 and 5 min
- D   They are not useful in intubated babies
- E   A blue baby scores 0

2.19 Features linked to depression in a child of 10 years may include:

- A   Diabetes mellitus
- B   Epilepsy
- C   Primary enuresis
- D   Abdominal pain
- E   Recent involvement in vandalism

2.20 With regard to developmental dysplasia of the hip:

- A   It is more common in boys
- B   It occurs in 5–20 per 1000 live births
- C   It affects the right hip more than the left
- D   The diagnosis should be confirmed by ultrasonography
- E   It is associated with a breech presentation

2.21 Features of cystic fibrosis include:

- A   Rectal prolapse
- B   Prolonged neonatal jaundice
- C   Digital clubbing
- D   Failure to thrive
- E   *Pseudomonas* chest infection

2.22 Roseola infantum:

○ A Presents with a rash on the first day
○ B Has an incubation period of approximately 5–15 days
○ C Is commonly the result of herpesvirus type 6
○ D Is also known as 'fifth disease'
○ E Is associated with pneumonia

2.23 Causes of tall stature include:

○ A Constitutional
○ B Homocystinuria
○ C Hyperthyroidism
○ D Pseudohypoparathyroidism
○ E Cushing syndrome

2.24 With regard to the treatment of asthma

○ A Aminophylline cannot be given if the child is already on regular oral theophylline
○ B Cromoglicate is a useful agent in the treatment of acute asthma
○ C Inhalers deliver less than 5% of the drug to the lungs
○ D The incidence of oral candidiasis can be reduced if steroids are inhaled via a spacer device
○ E Regular inhaled low-dose steroids do not result in growth retardation

2.25 Examples of primary prevention include:

○ A Cycling helmets
○ B Stair gates
○ C Teaching children road safety from a young age
○ D Smoke alarms
○ E Childproof catches on cupboards

questions

2.26 The Dubowitz system for assessment of gestational age include the following external criteria:

- A Nipple formation
- B Ear firmness
- C Nail development
- D Presence of eyelashes
- E Breast size

2.27 Infants born to mothers with poorly controlled diabetes may have:

- A Erb's palsy
- B Sacral agenesis
- C Hypomagnesaemia
- D Hypercalcaemia
- E Anaemia

2.28 With regard to the management of urinary tract infections (UTIs):

- A Amoxicillin is the first-line treatment in children
- B Prophylactic antibiotics are given four times daily for 1 month
- C It includes avoiding constipation
- D Asymptomatic bacteriuria should always be treated with appropriate antibiotics
- E It may involve surgery

2.29 Cerebral palsy:

- A Is a progressive condition
- B Has a prevalence of 2.5 in 1000
- C Is associated with a learning disability in 70–80% of cases
- D Is caused by perinatal hypoxic–ischaemic injury in most cases
- E May present with clumsiness

2.30 The stepwise treatment of asthma involves:

○ A Step 2: the regular use of low-dose inhaled steroids and bronchodilators as required

○ B Starting at 'step 1' and gradually stepping up treatment until an appropriate level is reached

○ C Step 4: the regular use of high-dose systemic steroids

○ D 'Stepping down' if control has been good for over 3 months

○ E Step 5: the addition of slow release xanthine, ± nebulised β agonist, ± alternate-day prednisolone, ± ipratropium or β-agonist subcutaneous infusion

2.31 With regard to the epidemiology of asthma:

○ A Asthma causes approximately 50 deaths per year in the UK

○ B Most deaths occur among 0–4 year olds

○ C Asthma affects 2–5% of all children in the UK

○ D The prevalence has gradually been decreasing over the past 20 years

○ E The mortality rate has gradually been decreasing over the past 10 years

2.32 Concerning cystic fibrosis:

○ A The gene for cystic fibrosis is located on the long arm of chromosome 7

○ B It may be diagnosed antenatally by chorionic villous sampling (CVS)

○ C The risk of two carriers having an affected child is 1 in 2

○ D It has a gene carrier rate of 1 in 40 in the white population

○ E Approximately 75–80% of cystic fibrosis gene mutations in the UK are caused by a deletion at ΔF508

questions

2.33 With respect to generalised 'absences':

- A They are more common in girls
- B They are associated with mental disability
- C Thirty per cent go on to develop generalised tonic–clonic epilepsy
- D The EEG shows unilateral spike waves over the rolandic area
- E First-line treatment is carbamazepine

2.34 Chronic constipation:

- A Often presents with diarrhoea
- B Is normal in breast-fed babies
- C Is frequently diet related
- D Is associated with Down's syndrome
- E Is defined as the infrequent passage of stools

2.35 With regard to case conferences for child abuse:

- A The Butler-Schloss report recommends that parents must always be invited to attend the case conference
- B They should ideally be held during the Emergency Protection Order (EPO)
- C The GP should be invited to attend
- D They have the capacity only to decide whether the child should be placed on the Child Protection Register
- E They must be attended by a senior officer from Social Services

EXTENDED MATCHING QUESTIONS

2.36 Theme: choice of investigations

- ○ A Blood cultures
- ○ B Bone marrow aspiration cytology
- ○ C Clotting screen
- ○ D C-reactive protein (CRP)
- ○ E Erythrocyte sedimentation rate (ESR)
- ○ F Full blood count (FBC)
- ○ G Glucose-6-phosphate dehydrogenase (G6PDH) assay
- ○ H Haemoglobin electrophoresis
- ○ I Monospot
- ○ J Peripheral blood film

For each of the following cases, please choose the investigation most likely to give a definitive diagnosis from the above list (each item may be used once or not at all):

1   A 6-month-old African–Caribbean infant presents with dactylitis.
2   A 7-year-old girl, who had an upper respiratory tract infection (URTI) 1 week ago, bruises easily and has developed petechiae.
3   A 14-year-old boy presents with a sore throat and palatal petechiae.

2.37 Theme: decisions about life-saving treatment

○ A The brain-dead child
○ B The 'no chance' situation
○ C The 'no purpose' situation
○ D The persistent vegetative state
○ E The 'unbearable' situation

For each of the following cases, please choose the most appropriate criterion under which life-saving treatment could be withdrawn (as identified by the Royal College of Paediatrics and Child Health [RCPCH]) from the above list (each item may be used once or not at all):

1 A 4-year-old girl who, despite maximal intensive care, is deteriorating as a result of meningococcal septicaemia.

2 A 5-year-old boy who has relapsed for the third time with acute myeloblastic leukaemia and doesn't wish for further chemotherapy.

3 A 1-year-old, who having sustained such severe head injuries in a road traffic accident that he is expected to be profoundly brain damaged, develops a pneumonia while in the paediatric intensive care unit (PICU).

2.38 Theme: heart defects

○ A   Aortic stenosis
○ B   Atrial septal defect (ASD)
○ C   Coarctation of the aorta
○ D   Ebstein's anomaly
○ E   Innocent (flow) murmur
○ F   Patent ductus arteriosus (PDA)
○ G   Pulmonary stenosis
○ H   Tetralogy of Fallot
○ I   Transposition of the great arteries (TGA)
○ J   Ventricular septal defect (VSD)

For each of the following sets of clinical findings, please choose the most likely diagnosis from the above list (each item may be used once or not at all):

1   A 3-year-old child presents to his GP with a febrile illness and is noted to have a soft ejection systolic murmur at the left sternal edge (LSE) only.

2   A 12-hour-old newborn baby, at her discharge check, is noted to have a pansystolic murmur heard all over the precordium. The femoral pulses are very easily palpable.

3   A baby girl is seen for the 8-week check and is noted to have an ejection systolic murmur best heard in the pulmonary area. The second heart sound does not vary with respiration. There is 1 cm hepatomegaly.

2.39 Theme: common infections

○ A Adenovirus
○ B β-Haemolytic streptococcus
○ C Coxsackie virus A16
○ D Epstein–Barr virus (EBV)
○ E Human herpesvirus 6
○ F *Mycoplasma pneumoniae*
○ G Parvovirus B19
○ H Poxvirus
○ I Rhinovirus
○ J Varicella-zoster virus

For each of the following scenarios, please choose the most likely underlying causative organism from the above list (each item may be used once or not at all):

1   A 12-year-old boy has a painful erythematous throat for which he is prescribed a broad-spectrum antibiotic. He represents the following day with a florid maculopapular rash all over his trunk.

2   A 3-year-old is at nursery and her mother notices that she is unwell, refusing foods, and has some vesicles on her palms and toes.

3   A 7-year-old boy presents with feeling unwell and has a macular rash all over his body. There are some 'target lesions' visible.

2.40 Theme: statistics and research methods

○ A Incidence
○ B Lag time
○ C Lead time
○ D Length bias
○ E Likelihood ratio
○ F Number needed to treat
○ G Paired cohort
○ H Prevalence
○ I Sensitivity
○ J Specificity

For each of the following definitions, please choose the word that applies to it from the above list (each item may be used once or not at all):

1 Interval between identification of a condition by screening and the development of symptoms.
2 Odds of a positive test result in an affected individual compared with that of a positive result in an unaffected individual.
3 Proportion of people unaffected by a condition correctly identified by a designated test.

2.41 Theme: immediate interventions

A Adenosine 50 µg/kg i.v.
B Amiodarone 5 mg/kg i.v.
C Asynchronous DC shock – 0.5 J/kg
D Asynchronous DC shock – 2 J/kg
E Asynchronous DC shock – 4 J/kg
F Atropine 20 µg/kg i.v.
G Lidocaine 1 mg/kg i.v.
H Sodium bicarbonate 4.2% 4 mL/kg i.v.
I Synchronous DC shock – 0.5 J/kg
J Vagal manoeuvres

For the cases below, please choose the most appropriate immediate intervention (airway and breathing can be assumed to be already managed) from the above list (each item may be used once or not at all):

1   A 3-year-old has the following trace: SVT (supraventricular tachycardia). Her capillary refill time (CRT) is 4 s and her O_2 saturations (SaO_2) are 92% in 5 L O_2 by mask.
2   A 15-year-old girl with a history of deliberate self-harm presents acutely unwell. ECG monitoring shows the following trace – VT (ventricular tachycardia). Her pulse is weak but present, CRT is 5 s, SaO_2 90% in 10 L O_2 by mask.
3   A 2-year-old child is brought in who was found unresponsive by her parents. She is being ventilated by bag–valve–mask by the paramedics. She is pulseless and has this rhythm on the monitor: VF (ventricular fibrillation).

2.42 Theme: neoplasms

- A Acute myeloblastic leukaemia (AML)
- B Acute lymphoid leukaemia (ALL)
- C Atrial myxoma
- D Ewing's sarcoma
- E Medulloblastoma
- F Neuroblastoma
- G Non-Hodgkin's lymphoma
- H Osteosarcoma
- I Rhabdomyosarcoma
- J Wilms' tumour

For each of the following cases, please choose the single most likely diagnosis from the above list (each item may be used once or not at all):

1   A 2-year-old presents with a 1-month history of lethargy, not being himself and bruising easily. He has hepatosplenomegaly and a full blood count (FBC) reveals: Hb 9.2 g/dL, white cell count (WCC) 2.3 × 10⁹/L, platelets (plts) 50 × 10⁹/L.

2   A 3-year-old boy has a large left flank mass and a trace of blood in his urine.

3   A 9-year-old boy presents with lethargy, shortness of breath and night sweats. On examination splenomegaly can be felt. There are no blast cells present on the blood film.

questions

2.43 Theme: antimicrobial therapy

- ○ A Intravenous benzylpenicillin
- ○ B Ceftriaxone 50 mg/kg i.v.
- ○ C Cefotaxime 100 mg/kg i.v.
- ○ D Oral amoxicillin
- ○ E Oral trimethoprim
- ○ F Intravenous flucloxacillin
- ○ G Intravenous cefotaxime 50 mg/kg
- ○ H Oral ciprofloxacin
- ○ I Oral clarithromycin
- ○ J Oral cefalexin

From the list above select the most appropriate antibiotic for each of the clinical scenarios below:

1   A 3-year-old child presents to A&E unwell, tachycardic and with an evolving purpuric rash.

2   A 2-day-old baby collapses on the postnatal ward with probable sepsis. His mother had grown group B streptococci on a high vaginal swab at 32 weeks.

3   A 7-year-old boy with cystic fibrosis develops a productive cough. He is not exhibiting any signs of respiratory distress and is systemically well.

BEST OF FIVE QUESTIONS

2.44 **Which of the following statements best describes the circumstances in which parents would be legally permitted to smack their child?**

- A Anywhere on the body, but not on the face
- B Anywhere on the body, but only after consideration (not in the heat of the moment)
- C Anywhere on the body, as long as only the hand is used and no mark is left
- D Anywhere on the body, except the face, but only in the home and not in public
- E Anywhere on the body, as long as any implement used does not leave a mark

2.45 **Which of the following is the best first-line step in management of a 5-year-old child who develops constipation after a viral illness?**

- A Dietary advice
- B Seven-day trial of lactulose (10 mL twice daily)
- C One glycerin suppository
- D Two stat phosphate enemas
- E Admission for administration of Klean-Prep

2.46 **A baby boy is noted to have hypospadias at the postnatal check. The meatus is situated ventrally and a chordee is noted. The most important piece of advice to give to the parents is:**

- A His adult sexual function should be normal
- B You must be careful when washing his penis
- C He must not be circumcised
- D He may require surgery in later childhood
- E Treat your baby as normal

2.47 A 15-year-old girl presents with a 2-month history of abdominal pain. She has had no fever and no other symptoms. Examination reveals 3 cm hepatomegaly and splenomegaly. The single most useful investigation would be:

- A CRP
- B Blood film
- C Abdominal ultrasonography
- D Paul Bunnell test
- E Liver function tests (LFTs) + amylase

2.48 A child who has a 2-day history of fever has a bright-red, infected, left tympanic membrane. The child is eating and drinking well. What would be the most appropriate course of action?

- A Referral to ENT (ear, nose, throat) surgeon as an emergency
- B Referral to ENT surgeon as an outpatient
- C 5-day course of oral phenoxymethylpenicillin
- D Advice to parents that this is a self-limiting condition and is best left alone
- E Regular antipyretics and analgesics with review in 48 h

2.49 Which of the following is the likeliest pathology on a cranial ultrasonography performed on day 1 of the life of a pre-term baby born at 25 weeks' gestation?

- A Hydrocephalus
- B Gyral pattern
- C Periventricular leukomalacia
- D Intraventricular haemorrhage
- E Cerebral atrophy

2.50 What is the most important investigation to perform in a 3-week-old newborn baby boy who is feeding well and thriving, but is referred with jaundice?

○ A Direct and indirect bilirubin
○ B Thyroid function tests (TFTs)
○ C LFTs
○ D Urine organic acids
○ E Coombs' test

2.51 An 8-month-old infant presents to A&E with a 3-day history of frequent watery diarrhoea and vomiting. On examination she is 5% dehydrated. She is refusing to drink in A&E. Which of the following is the most appropriate course of action?

○ A Admit for intravenous rehydration (maintenance and 5% deficit)
○ B Observe for 4 h in A&E; if she tolerates oral fluids discharge her; if not admit for intravenous rehydration
○ C Admit for enteral rehydration via a nasogastric tube
○ D Admit for intravenous rehydration (maintenance) + oral fluids as tolerated
○ E Short course of oral cefalexin

2.52 In a mother who is hepatitis B surface antibody (HBsAb) positive and core antigen (HBeAg) positive, which of the following combinations is the most appropriate for her newborn baby?

○ A Hepatitis B vaccine
○ B Hepatitis B immunoglobulin
○ C Hepatitis B vaccine and hepatitis B immunoglobulin
○ D Hepatitis B vaccine and intravenous pooled immunoglobulin
○ E Hepatitis B and hepatitis C vaccines combined

2.53 Which of the following social milestones would you expect a normally developing 15-month-old infant to have most recently acquired?

- ○ A Brush teeth with help
- ○ B Play ball with examiner
- ○ C Wave bye-bye
- ○ D Put on T-shirt with no help
- ○ E Play 'pat-a-cake'

2.54 In primary nocturnal enuresis in a 5-year-old, which of the following is the most appropriate initial management strategy?

- ○ A Family counselling
- ○ B Star chart
- ○ C Verbal chastisement
- ○ D Short trial of imipramine
- ○ E Short trial of desmopressin

2.55 Which of the following gross motor milestones would you expect 90% of normally developing children to have most recently developed by 4 years?

- ○ A Able to run steadily
- ○ B Walk backwards
- ○ C Hop on one leg
- ○ D Walk up stairs unaided
- ○ E Throw ball over-hand

2.56 A 4-year-old girl is suffering physical abuse at home. Which of the following interventions would be most appropriate to apply if her welfare is thought to be in immediate danger?

A Police Protection Order (PPO)
B Emergency Protection Order
C Court wardship
D Section 47 meeting
E Temporary foster placement

2.57 A 4-year-old girl suffers a femoral fracture in a road traffic accident. She also has a contusion on her right forehead. She is screaming with the pain from her leg. Which of the following would be the most effective and safest form of analgesia?

A Per rectum (p.r.) diclofenac and oral codeine
B Splinting of the fractured limb
C Paracetamol, ibuprofen and codeine per os (p.o.)
D Morphine intravenously
E Femoral nerve block

2.58 Which of the following diagnoses is the most likely in a 3-year-old boy who has epilepsy and, on examination, has numerous depigmented macules and two café-au-lait spots?

A Tuberous sclerosis
B Neurofibromatosis 1
C Ataxia telangiectasia
D Incontinentia pigmenti
E Sturge–Weber syndrome

2.59 A 2-year-old white boy is diagnosed with nephrotic syndrome. Which of the following is the most likely underlying pathology?

○ A Minimal change disease
○ B Mesangial proliferative disease
○ C Focal segmental glomerular sclerosis
○ D 'Finnish'-type microcystic disease
○ E Cystinosis

2.60 A 4-year-old child presents with coryzal symptoms, cough, fever and abdominal pain. There is no dysuria and the urine dipstick is unremarkable. On examination the pain is in the left upper quadrant but is not severe. Which is the most likely cause?

○ A UTI
○ B Appendicitis
○ C Pyelonephritis
○ D Left basal chest infection
○ E Mesenteric adenitis

2.61 A 6-week-old baby is referred for back arching and crying. He possets after feeds, especially when he lies on his back. He is thriving. You suspect gastro-oesophageal reflux (GOR). What is the most appropriate course of action?

○ A Barium swallow
○ B Trial of Gaviscon
○ C Trial of domperidone and ranitidine
○ D Reassure the parents
○ E A pH study

2.62 A 15-year-old girl is referred after a deliberate paracetamol overdose. She reports having taken five pills 45 min ago. What is the most appropriate course of action?

○ A Administer activated charcoal and take paracetamol levels at 4 h

○ B Administer activated charcoal and start intravenous N-acetylcysteine, then take paracetamol levels at 4 h

○ C Start intravenous N-acetylcysteine, and take levels at 4 h

○ D Wait and take blood at 4 h for paracetamol levels

○ E Discharge her because it is not a harmful dose.

2.63 The 15-year-old girl in Question 2.62 has paracetamol levels well below the treatment line at 4 h. She says she only took the pills as a 'cry for help' and regrets doing it. What is the most appropriate course of action?

○ A Discharge her with an urgent child psychiatry outpatient appointment

○ B Discharge her and contact the school educational psychologist

○ C Admit her for formal assessment by a child psychiatrist

○ D Admit her for observation overnight and discharge her if well the next day with a child psychiatry outpatient appointment

○ E Discharge her for GP follow-up

2.64 A 22-month-old boy is seen because there are concerns about his motor development. He sat unsupported at 10 months, crawled at 1 year and started to walk unsupported at 20 months. His social, language and fine motor development appear age appropriate. Which of the following investigations would be the most useful?

- A   Detailed physiotherapy assessment
- B   TFTs
- C   Creatine kinase (CK) level
- D   Cranial MRI (magnetic resonance imaging)
- E   Electromyogram (EMG)

2.65 A diagnosis of Henoch–Schönlein purpura (HSP) is made in a 7-year-old child. There is a trace of blood on a urine dipstick. His blood pressure is normal. There is mild arthralgia controlled with ibuprofen and paracetamol. What is the most appropriate course of action?

- A   Referral for renal biopsy
- B   Weekly blood pressure and urine dipsticks until clear
- C   Discharge from follow-up
- D   Weekly serum urea and electrolytes (U&Es)
- E   Monthly outpatient clinic appointments for 6 months

2.66 A previously well 8-year-old boy presents to A&E with a mild fever and painful swelling of his right wrist and left ankle, his right ankle having been affected the previous week. Twenty days ago he had tonsillitis. On examination his temperature is 38°C, respiration 30/min, pulse 120/min, blood pressure (BP) 80 mmHg systolic, capillary refill 2 s. He has normal heart sounds, a significant cardiac murmur and a pericardial rub, but no palpable liver. His CRP is 150 mg/L and his ECG shows a slightly prolonged P–R interval. Of the following, the most appropriate treatment is:

   A Low-dose aspirin

   B Intravenous flucloxacillin

   C Diuretics

   D Bed rest

   E ACTH (adrenocorticotrophic hormone)

2.67 A 3-year-old is brought to A&E having been found with an empty pill bottle of his grandmother's. There is no information as to what the tablets were. On examination he is drowsy, pale and sweaty. His respiratory rate (RR) is 40/min, his BP 70/30 mmHg and his pulse 170/min and very thready. Which of the following drugs were the tablets most likely to have been?

   A β Blockers

   B Aspirin

   C Paracetamol

   D Iron

   E Tricyclic antidepressant (TCA)

2.68 A 12-year-old boy complains of excessive tiredness and fatigue at any time of day. He has missed a lot of school over the past 6 months and says he can't concentrate. He complains of headaches, aching limbs and variable appetite. He stays at home most of the time and his mother has had to give up work to look after him. On examination, he seems quiet but not clinically depressed. A detailed general and neurological examination reveals no abnormalities. His FBC, CRP, LFTs, U&Es, T_4 (thyroxine) and urinalysis are normal. The most relevant management is:

A Arrange regular physiotherapy

B Prescribe supplemental iron and vitamins

C Encourage bed rest every morning

D Prescribe fluoxetine

E Organise home tuition

PAPER 3

3.1 Concerning secretory otitis media (glue ear):

- A It can cause a sensorineural hearing loss
- B It may present as a behavioural problem
- C The primary role of the grommet is to drain the middle-ear effusion
- D Most grommets require surgical removal
- E Most affected children will have normal hearing by 8 years of age

3.2 In *Haemophilus influenzae* type b (Hib) disease:

- A Sixty per cent of invasive Hib disease presents as meningitis
- B The mortality rate for Hib meningitis is approximately 20%
- C Hib infection is rare before 2 years of age
- D Hib immunisation is contraindicated in HIV-positive individuals
- E All infants in the absence of genuine contraindications should be immunised at 2, 3 and 4 months of age

questions

3.3 **With regard to paediatric resuscitation:**

- A Most cardiac arrests in children are the result of respiratory arrest
- B A Breslow tape is of no use
- C Cardiac arrest secondary to drowning has a particularly poor prognosis
- D Intraosseous access is suitable for children aged up to 6 years
- E A cuffed endotracheal tube should always be used to prevent regurgitation and aspiration

3.4 **With regard to growth charts:**

- A Infants aged 0–1 year should have at least three recordings of height and weight
- B All children below the 2nd centile for height should be reviewed by the GP
- C All children below the 1st centile for height should be referred for a specialist opinion
- D Normal growth velocity of children over 2 years of age is 10 cm/year
- E Children with a growth velocity less than the 25th or greater than the 75th centile should be referred for a specialist opinion

3.5 **Signs of child abuse include:**

- A 'Frozen watchfulness'
- B Acute hyphaema
- C A single green/yellow bruise over the forehead of a toddler
- D A mid-clavicular fracture in a 10-day-old newborn
- E Scalds over both buttocks

3.6 **With regard to dermatophyte (ringworm) infections in children:**

○ A Tinea pedis is rare in children aged under 5 years
○ B *Trichophyton* sp. often causes tinea capitis
○ C Tinea corporis typically presents with hair loss, and circular patches of alopecia with scaling skin and broken hairs
○ D These are caused by superficial filamentous (hyphae) fungal infections of the skin, which fluoresce under Wood's light
○ E Large infected areas may require a 2-week course of oral griseofulvin

3.7 **Risk factors for developmental dysplasia of the hip (DDH) include:**

○ A Male sex
○ B Oligohydramnios
○ C Sister had DDH
○ D Forceps delivery
○ E Maternal drug abuse

3.8 **Signs of severe acute asthma include:**

○ A Normal $Paco_2$ on arterial blood gas analysis
○ B Agitation
○ C Use of accessory muscles
○ D Presence of pectus carinatum
○ E Pulsus paradoxus of 10–20 mmHg

questions

3.9   With regard to acute epiglottitis:

○   A   It commonly occurs in infants aged less than 1 year
○   B   The incidence has significantly decreased since the
         introduction of the Hib vaccine
○   C   It is associated with septicaemia
○   D   The child characteristically holds the head in hyperflexion
○   E   It should be confirmed by a lateral neck radiograph

3.10   Known side effects of phenytoin include:

○   A   Megaloblastic anaemia
○   B   Lymphoma
○   C   Dyskinesia (including choreoathetosis)
○   D   Systemic lupus erythematosus (SLE)
○   E   Gum hypertrophy

3.11   With regard to tics:

○   A   They are defined as stereotypical, repetitive, voluntary
         movements
○   B   Simple developmental tics affect 15% of primary age
         schoolchildren (Years 1–6)
○   C   They are generally not of pathological significance and are
         usually outgrown by age 4 years
○   D   They may be manifestations of tension or emotional
         disorder when they commonly persist beyond adolescence
○   E   They may be familial

3.12 With regard to childhood asthma:

A Dehydration is common in asthma, so intravenous fluids should be increased to one-third above normal maintenance in severe cases

B A chest radiograph on admission should be taken in all children presenting with an acute exacerbation

C Peak expiratory flow rate (PEFR) should be measured in children older than 5 years

D In the UK the most common reason for a child to be admitted to hospital is for an acute exacerbation of asthma

E Intravenous steroids are first-line treatment in all cases of acute exacerbation of asthma

3.13 The MMR vaccine:

A Is contraindicated in patients allergic to neomycin

B Should not be given within 3 weeks of another live vaccine (except oral polio vaccine [Sabin])

C Is safe in pregnancy

D Commonly results in a rash with or without fever from day 5 to day 10, lasting approximately 2 days

E Is contraindicated in patients who have received an injection of immunoglobulin within 3 months

3.14 Maternal risk factors for increased perinatal mortality and morbidity include:

A Age between 16 and 35 years

B Short stature

C A birth interval of 18–36 months

D A twin pregnancy

E A previous ectopic pregnancy

3.15 Plagiocephaly:

○ A Is often associated with babies who are consistently put into the cot on the same side

○ B May present with torticollis at age 6 months to 3 years

○ C Is associated with craniosynostosis

○ D Has an increased incidence of epilepsy

○ E Generally spontaneously improves with time

3.16 Known side effects of carbamazepine include:

○ A Aplastic anaemia

○ B Rickets

○ C Ataxia

○ D Transient hair loss

○ E Rash

3.17 Known side effects of clonazepam include:

○ A Salivary and bronchial hypersecretion

○ B Nystagmus

○ C Somnolence and hypotonia

○ D Reversible leukopenia

○ E Acne

3.18 Cystic fibrosis:

○ A Affects approximately 1 in 2000 live births in the UK

○ B Has an X-linked inheritance

○ C May present with meconium ileus

○ D Is associated with delayed puberty

○ E Is associated with nasal polyposis

3.19 Causes of haematuria include:

○ A Exercise
○ B Idiopathic
○ C Allergy
○ D Meatal stenosis
○ E Malaria

3.20 Examples of secondary prevention include:

○ A Seat belts
○ B Blister packs for prescription drugs
○ C Teaching parents first aid skills
○ D Fire extinguishers kept in the house
○ E Speed limits

3.21 Congenital rubella syndrome includes:

○ A Deafness
○ B Microphthalmia
○ C Cardiac defects
○ D Cerebral palsy
○ E Saddle nose

3.22 With regard to congenital heart disease (CHD):

○ A Down's syndrome is associated with an increased incidence of ventricular septal defect (VSD) and atrial septal defect (ASD)
○ B It has an incidence of approximately 8 per 10 000 live births
○ C An indometacin infusion can be used to keep the ductus arteriosus patent until corrective surgery can be carried out
○ D VSD is the most common congenital heart defect
○ E The incidence of cyanotic CHD is approximately three times that of acyanotic lesions

65

3.23 With regard to foster care:

- A Short-term fostering is usually up to 18 months
- B Long-term fostering is preferred for younger children
- C It is more likely to be successful if there are children of a similar age in the placement family
- D There is usually a limit of three foster children per family
- E Children in long-term foster care require a 6-monthly medical examination

3.24 In the treatment of asthma

- A Oral salbutamol syrup is useful in the treatment of infants and toddlers
- B A plastic coffee cup may be used as a spacer device
- C Inhaled drugs cannot be effectively delivered to children aged under 2 years
- D A 3-year-old can use dry powder inhalers
- E A spacer device is unsuitable in children aged over 10 years

3.25 Risk factors for sudden infant death syndrome (SIDS) include:

- A Female sex
- B Twins
- C Bottle-feeding
- D Previous history of a sibling dying from SIDS
- E Supine sleeping position

3.26 Common features of cystic fibrosis include:

- A Anorexia
- B Steatorrhoea
- C A positive sweat test, where the concentration of sweat sodium is > 70 mmol/L
- D An increased incidence in Chinese people
- E Male impotence

3.27 With regard to vesicoureteric reflux (VUR):

A It should be routinely screened for in all children aged under 5 years

B Ten per cent of children with VUR will develop renal scarring

C Grade II VUR involves urine refluxing into the kidney on micturition only

D If severe it may require an endoscopic, submucosal, Teflon injection

E It requires monitoring with serial ultrasonography

3.28 With regard to spastic hemiplegia:

A The legs are more severely affected than the arms

B It may result from an infarct of the cortex or internal capsule

C Almost all affected children walk by school age

D One leg may be shorter than the other

E It characteristically results in learning difficulties

3.29 Signs of sexual abuse in children include:

A HIV infection

B Clitoromegaly

C Sexualised behaviour inappropriate for age

D Anal fissures

E Anal skin tags

3.30 With regard to acute renal failure (ARF):

A Gentamicin is a cause of prerenal failure

B It may be caused by haemolytic uraemic syndrome

C It may be complicated by convulsions or tetany

D Management should include a high-protein diet

E An indication for dialysis is a plasma urea > 54 mmol/L

3.31 Signs of severe acute asthma include:

◯ A Presence of a loud wheeze

◯ B Being too breathless to eat

◯ C Heart rate between 100 and 140 beats/min

◯ D PEFR < 50% of predicted

◯ E Respiratory rate > 50 breaths/min

3.32 With regard to infantile colic:

◯ A It characteristically presents with paroxysmal crying and 'pulling up' of the legs

◯ B It peaks between 3 and 6 months

◯ C It can be caused by cows' milk protein intolerance

◯ D There is no effective medical treatment

◯ E It may require hospital admission

3.33 With regard to a urinary tract infection (UTI):

◯ A It is more common in boys in the first month of life

◯ B *Escherichia coli* is responsible in approximately 80% of cases

◯ C Most UTIs are haematogenous in origin in neonates

◯ D Significant bacteriuria occurs with > 103 CFU (colony-forming units) of bacteria/mL

◯ E VUR is found in approximately 35% of children with a UTI

3.34 With regard to generalised tonic–clonic epilepsy:

◯ A Onset is generally after 5 years of age

◯ B It is not associated with an aura

◯ C The EEG may be normal between seizures

◯ D After 15 years approximately 80% remain 'fit free' off treatment

◯ E First-line treatment is carbamazepine

3.35 Non-accidental injury (NAI) should be suspected if:

○   A   Parents attend A&E immediately
○   B   Parents are over-protective
○   C   A fractured tibia is seen in a 6-month-old infant
○   D   The child has a depressed skull fracture
○   E   The child has bilateral black eyes

questions

questions

EXTENDED MATCHING QUESTIONS

3.36 Theme: respiratory distress in the newborn

○ A Congenital cystic adenomatous malformation
○ B Congenital diaphragmatic hernia
○ C Congenital pneumonia
○ D Meconium aspiration syndrome
○ E Persistent pulmonary hypertension of the newborn
○ F Pneumothorax
○ G Pulmonary haemorrhage
○ H Pulmonary hypoplasia
○ I Surfactant deficient lung disease (hyaline membrane disease)
○ J Transient tachypnoea of the newborn

For each of the following scenarios, please choose the most likely diagnosis from the above list (each item may be used once or not at all):

1   An infant born at 24 weeks' gestation who has respiratory distress at birth.
2   An infant born at 33 weeks' gestation with profound respiratory distress. Antenatal history reveals that there was rupture of the membranes at 16 weeks, and the mother has been on erythromycin.
3   A baby born by elective caesarean section at term (for breech presentation) after an uncomplicated pregnancy. At 15 min of age the baby is noted to be grunting.

3.37 Theme: genetic diseases

○ A Autosomal dominant
○ B Autosomal dominant with incomplete penetrance
○ C Autosomal recessive
○ D Autosomal recessive with incomplete penetrance
○ E Lionised X linked
○ F Robertsonian translocation
○ G Sporadic
○ H Uniparental disomy
○ I X-linked dominant
○ J X-linked recessive

For each of the following conditions, please choose the most appropriate mode of inheritance from the above list (each item may be used once or not at all):

1 Achondroplasia.
2 Sickle cell disease.
3 Duchenne muscular dystrophy.

3.38 Theme: blood disorders

○ A Acute lymphoblastic leukaemia
○ B Aplastic anaemia
○ C β-Thalassaemia intermedia
○ D Christmas disease
○ E G6PDH (glucose-6-phosphate dehydrogenase) deficiency
○ F Haemophilia A
○ G Henoch–Schönlein purpura
○ H Immune-mediated thrombocytopenia purpura
○ I Meningococcal septicaemia
○ J Sickle cell disease

For each of the following cases please choose the diagnosis that best fits the clinical and laboratory information from the above list (each item may be used once or not at all):

1   A 4-year-child of eastern Mediterranean origin presents pale and tired after a UTI treated with antibiotics. His full blood count (FBC) reveals Hb 4.2 g/dL, white cell count (WCC) 12 × 10^9/L, platelets (plts) 332 × 10^9/L, reticulocytes 6%.

2   A 6-year-old child develops a petechial rash. Her FBC shows Hb 11 g/dL, WCC 2.4 × 10^9/L, plts 9 × 10^9/L. A bone marrow trephine shows an increase in megakaryocytes.

3   A 9-year-old child is febrile but well, and develops a purpuric rash on his lower limbs. His FBC shows Hb 13 g/dL, WCC 12 × 10^9/L (neutrophils 2 × 10^9/L, lymphocytes 10 × 10^9/L), plts 540 × 10^9/L. Coagulation profile: international normalised ratio (INR) 1.2, activated partial thromboplastin time (APTT) 28 s, prothrombin time (PT) 11 s.

questions

3.39 Theme: infant nutrition

- ○ A 2 months
- ○ B 4 months
- ○ C 7 months
- ○ D 9 months
- ○ E 1 year
- ○ F 18 months
- ○ G 2 years
- ○ H 3 years
- ○ I 4 years
- ○ J 5 years

For each of the following foodstuffs, please choose the most appropriate age for their introduction (in a normal infant) from the above list (each item may be used once or not at all):

1. Pasta.
2. Baby rice.
3. Pureed meat and vegetables.

3.40 Theme: systemic diseases

- ○ A Behçet's disease
- ○ B Dermatomyositis
- ○ C Kawasaki's disease
- ○ D Lyme disease
- ○ E Pauciarticular juvenile idiopathic arthritis
- ○ F Polyarticular juvenile idiopathic arthritis
- ○ G Rheumatic fever
- ○ H Septic arthritis
- ○ I Still's disease
- ○ J SLE

For each of the following case scenarios, please choose the most likely diagnosis from the above list (each item may be used once or not at all):

1   A 3-year-old boy has had a fever for 6 days, swollen hands, conjunctivitis and cracked lips. Investigation reveals: C-reactive protein (CRP) 67 mg/L, erythrocyte sedimentation rate (ESR) 40 mm, Hb 12.1 g/dL, WCC 16 × 10^9/L (neutrophils 7 × 10^9/L, lymphocytes 8 × 10^9/L), plts 480 × 10^9/L.

2   A 12-year-old girl presents with feeling unwell, lethargy and pain in her knees and legs. On examination she is febrile (37.7°C), and has an erythematous rash on the face, particularly the eyelids. Investigations show: ESR 50 mm, normal FBC, creatine kinase (CK) 700 IU/L.

3   A 7-year-old girl presents with pain in both knees, left ankle and right wrist. On examination, the joints involved are swollen, tender and have limitation of range of movement. Investigations show CRP 35 g/dL, anti-neutrophil antibody (ANA) positive, rheumatoid factor negative, dsDNA antibodies negative, anti-streptolysin O test (ASOT) negative.

3.41 Theme: syndromes

- ○ A Achondroplasia
- ○ B Beckwith–Wiedemann syndrome
- ○ C Down's syndrome
- ○ D Fragile X syndrome
- ○ E Noonan syndrome
- ○ F Patau syndrome
- ○ G Pierre Robin syndrome
- ○ H Prader–Willi syndrome
- ○ I Rubenstein–Taybi syndrome
- ○ J Turner's syndrome

For each of the following cases, please choose the diagnosis that best fits with the clinical features from the above list (each item may be used once or not at all):

1   A term baby is noted to have a cleft palate and small chin. She appears to have problems breathing when placed supine.

2   A 4-year-old boy is having problems keeping up academically with his peers. On examination his neck is mildly webbed and he has low-set ears.

3   A 6-year-old boy has marked behavioural problems. On examination he has large ears and a high forehead.

3.42 Theme: immunisations

○ A Acellular pertussis vaccine
○ B Conjugate pneumococcal vaccine
○ C Hepatitis A vaccine
○ D Hepatitis B Vaccine
○ E Influenza vaccine
○ F Palivizumab (anti-RSV [respiratory syncytial virus] immunoglobulin)
○ G Ribavirin
○ H Salk polio vaccine
○ I Single measles vaccine
○ J Unconjugated pneumococcal vaccine

For the following situations please choose one vaccine that should be used instead of, or in addition to, the routine scheduled vaccines from the above list (each item may be used once or not at all):

1 An ex-premature baby is discharged in October with home oxygen. He has had the first three sets of the universal schedule (while an inpatient).
2 A 4-year-old whose sibling is receiving chemotherapy for AML.
3 A 3-year-old infant has a splenectomy after a road traffic accident.

3.43 Theme: drugs

○ A Intravenous aciclovir
○ B Per os fluconazole
○ C Intravenous ribavirin
○ D Intravenous ganciclovir
○ E Per os azithromycin
○ F Intravenous vancomycin
○ G Intravenous flucloxacillin
○ H Intravenous co-amoxiclav
○ I Intravenous cefotaxime
○ J Intravenous amphotericin

For each of the clinical scenarios below select, from the list above, the most appropriate therapeutic agent.

1 A 12-year-old presents with cough, fever and feeling unwell. Her saturations are 98% in air and her respiratory rate is 24/min without recession. There are diffuse crackles throughout her lung fields on auscultation

2 A 2-year-old child presents with a 2-day history of headache and mood change. She is febrile. She has a focal seizure with secondary generalisation in A&E. Computed tomography (CT) shows changes in the temporal lobe.

3 An 18-month-old child is admitted with infected eczema affecting both elbows, the chest and behind the left knee. He is febrile (38°C).

BEST OF FIVE QUESTIONS

3.44 A 9-month-old infant presents with vomiting and crying. On examination she is afebrile and has a diffusely tender abdomen. No masses are palpable. Which one of the following diagnoses is the most important to exclude?

○ A Gastroenteritis
○ B Intussusception
○ C Mesenteric adenitis
○ D Hirschsprung's disease
○ E Colic

3.45 A 9-month-old infant presents with coryzal symptoms and a hoarse barking cough. Select the most likely causative agent from the list below.

○ A Adenovirus
○ B *Haemophilus influenzae* type b
○ C Parainfluenza virus type 3
○ D Parvovirus
○ E *Corynebacterium* species

3.46 A 7-week-old baby boy is referred with a 2-week history of vomiting. He is being formula fed 5 oz (approximately 150 mL) every 2–3 h. On examination he is well, thriving and has a normal examination. The most likely diagnosis is:

○ A Pyloric stenosis
○ B Gastro-oesophageal reflux
○ C Over-feeding
○ D Gastroenteritis
○ E Jejunal stenosis

3.47 Which of the following is the first sign of puberty in boys?

- ○ A Growth spurt
- ○ B Pubic hair development
- ○ C Deepening of the voice
- ○ D Increase in testicular volume
- ○ E Axillary hair development

3.48 You diagnose a 7-year-old girl as having a generalised chest infection. Her respiratory rate is 30/min, SaO_2 98% in air; there is no recession. What would be the most appropriate course of action?

- ○ A Admit for intravenous antibiotics
- ○ B Allow home but arrange for intravenous antibiotics to be given by the home care nurses
- ○ C A 7-day course of oral amoxicillin
- ○ D A 7-day course of oral erythromycin
- ○ E Admit for oral antibiotics

3.49 A 3-year-old, fully immunised child presents with fever and difficulty in breathing. She has had tonsillitis over the past week. On examination she looks unwell, has mild recession and a soft stridor is audible. What is the most likely diagnosis?

- ○ A Retropharyngeal abscess
- ○ B Bacterial tracheitis
- ○ C Epiglottitis
- ○ D Severe croup
- ○ E Fulminant pneumonia

3.50 A 13-year-old girl attends her GP surgery wanting to be prescribed the oral contraceptive pill (OCP). She is sexually active but does not want her mother to know (despite reasoning). Which of the following would be the most appropriate course of action?

A Refusal to prescribe because she is under the age of informed consent

B Prescribe her the OCP because it would be in her best interests

C Prescribe her the OCP if she meets the Gillick criteria

D Prescribe her the OCP on the condition that she gets parental consent

E Refuse to prescribe because this would condone under-age sexual intercourse, which is illegal

3.51 A 18-month-old infant who has an upper respiratory tract infection (URTI) presents with a convulsion. Which of the following features best fits with a typical febrile convulsion?

A One minute of left arm shaking followed by 6 min of tonic–clonic movement of all four limbs

B Eyes rolling back followed by a 3-min generalised tonic–clonic seizure; drowsy afterwards for 1 h

C Going vacant and unresponsive for 2 min; back to normal self afterwards

D A 25-min generalised tonic–clonic seizure terminated with intravenous lorazepam

E A 5-min generalised tonic–clonic seizure; drowsy afterwards then a further 15-min generalised tonic–clonic seizure

3.52 **You are called to counsel a woman in premature labour at 23/40. Which of the following is the most appropriate information to give initially?**

○ A Unfortunately at this gestation there is a 10–20% survival rate, and of the survivors 50% will have some degree of handicap

○ B Unfortunately at this gestation there are the following survival and handicap statistics (tell her the figures for your own unit)

○ C Survival at this gestation is generally poor, and survivors may have long-term problems (then discuss with her the option of not resuscitating if the baby is in a poor condition)

○ D Babies at this gestation are very immature and will have a long and difficult time in the neonatal intensive care (then discuss the likely problems and interventions that may be necessary)

○ E Babies at this gestation are extremely early and often do not survive but we will do everything we can

3.53 **Which of the following language milestones would you expect a normally developing 2-year-old child to have most recently acquired?**

○ A Six-word vocabulary
○ B More than 100-word vocabulary
○ C Three-word phrases
○ D Tuneful babbling
○ E Singing nursery rhymes

3.54 A 2-day-old neonate of 28 weeks' gestation has a right-sided intraventricular haemorrhage with no ventricular dilatation while on the ventilator. Which of the following is the best advice to give to the parents?

○ A There are likely to be no significant long-term effects

○ B There should be no significant long-term effects provided that the ventricle doesn't dilate

○ C There may be some mild impairment of the left arm/leg

○ D There may be some very mild concentration difficulties in childhood

○ E It is probable that there will be no significant long-term effects but his development will be closely followed just in case

3.55 A 13-year-old boy develops gynaecomastia and comes to you because he is concerned. He reveals that he is being bullied at school as a result. What is the most appropriate course of action?

○ A Referral to a paediatric surgeon for consideration of surgical reduction of the breast tissue

○ B Arrange for assessment of the hypothalamic–pituitary axis

○ C Reassure him that this is physiological and a normal part of puberty

○ D Reassure him and arrange for clinical psychology support

○ E Reassure him and contact the school (with his consent) about the bullying

3.56 Which of the following is the most appropriate treatment for the contacts of a child who is admitted with meningococcal sepsis?

◯ A Treat all family members with rifampicin
◯ B Treat close contacts with rifampicin
◯ C Treat those contacts as advised by the Consultant for Communicable Disease Control (CCDC)
◯ D Treat close contacts: children with penicillin and adults with rifampicin
◯ E Leave the contact tracing and treatment to the CCDC

3.57 Which of the following is the best method of vascular access in a 5-year-old child brought into A&E in asystole?

◯ A Peripheral venous cannulation
◯ B Femoral venous central line insertion
◯ C Long saphenous venous cannulation
◯ D External jugular central line insertion
◯ E Tibial intraosseous needle insertion

3.58 A 2-year-old presents with a very painful scrotum. On examination the scrotum is swollen and inflamed on the right side. The testis on the right is not swollen although it is tender at the upper pole. What is the most likely diagnosis?

◯ A Testicular torsion
◯ B Idiopathic scrotal oedema
◯ C Torted hydatid of Morgagni
◯ D Epididymo-orchitis
◯ E Mumps orchitis

3.59 A 6-year-old complains that his foreskin balloons when he passes urine. On examination you note non-retractile foreskin with some preputial adhesions. What is the best course of action?

○ A Advise gentle retraction of the foreskin in the bath
○ B Advise that it can be normal at this age and should be left alone
○ C Advise applying 1% hydrocortisone cream twice daily for 1 week
○ D Refer for circumcision
○ E Send a preputial skin swab for microscopy, culture and sensitivity

3.60 A 7-year-old girl has had two generalised tonic–clonic seizures (each lasting 7 min). The EEG shows epileptiform activity. Which of the following is the most appropriate first-line anticonvulsant?

○ A Phenytoin
○ B Carbamazepine
○ C Lamotrigine
○ D Per rectum diazepam (p.r.n.)
○ E Sodium valproate

questions

3.61 An 18-month-old girl with eczema is on the following treatment regimen: Oilatum in baths; 'baby' shampoo and soap; aqueous cream to affected areas four times daily. Mother uses 'non-biological' washing powder. On examination her skin is erythematous, excoriated and lichenified over the knees, thighs and flexor surfaces of the elbows. Which of the following would be the next best step?

- A Use aqueous cream instead of soap; advise using a greasier emollient and try an antihistamine at night
- B Use 1% hydrocortisone to affected areas and continue with other measures
- C Use emollient wet wraps at night for 1 week then continue current treatment
- D Use fusidic acid–hydrocortisone on the affected areas for 1 week, then continue the current regimen
- E Advise mother to continue the current treatment and try to exclude dairy products from the diet

3.62 An 8-month-old infant had a confirmed UTI at age 5 months and is currently on prophylactic antibiotics. Renal ultrasonography at the time of the UTI showed left renal pelvicalyceal dilatation. What is the most appropriate investigation to perform next?

- A Repeat renal tract ultrasonography
- B Micturating cystourethrogram
- C DMSA (^{99m}Tc-dimercaptosuccinic acid) scan
- D MAG-3 (Mercapto Acetyl Tri Glycine) scan
- E Repeat urine for MC&S (microscopy, culture and sensitivity)

3.63 **A 9-year-old child has a large, swollen, fluctuant, left submandibular lymph node. You notice that there is gross caries in most of her teeth. There is a buccal swelling adjacent to her lower left 'E' (primary molar). What is the best course of action?**

○ A Course of oral amoxicillin and metronidazole and referral to her general dental practitioner (GDP)

○ B Admission for intravenous amoxicillin and metronidazole

○ C Referral to maxillofacial surgery for incision and drainage (I&D)

○ D Trial of oral antibiotics and surgical referral if no improvement after 5 days

○ E Course for 5 days of intravenous ceftriaxone administered at home by community nurses, with review after the course

3.64 **A 5-year-old boy has a history of recurrent nocturnal cough and frequent difficulty in breathing on exercise. He has recently been admitted with moderately severe wheeze that responded to nebulised bronchodilator therapy and a dose of oral prednisolone. What do you prescribe on discharge?**

○ A A home nebuliser with salbutamol as needed

○ B Becotide 200 μg twice daily via a metered dose inhaler (MDI)

○ C Flixotide 100 μg twice daily via a low-volume spacer

○ D Budesonide 200 μg twice daily via a dry powder device

○ E Montelukast 5 mg at night

questions

3.65 A 7-year-old boy with severe cerebral palsy and developmental delay was referred for investigation because of uncontrolled seizures and respiratory problems, initially diagnosed and treated as asthma. He attends a special school. He is a 'difficult feeder', and had clinical evidence of a chest infection on admission. He was noted to have recurrent spasmodic movements with arching of the back, throwing the arms and head and lurching forward. These were associated with gurgling noises in the throat but no loss of awareness. These were more frequent during respiratory illnesses and especially during or immediately after meals. Two EEGs were reported as normal. Antiepileptic drugs have had no significant effect. The clinical picture is most compatible with:

A Dystonic cerebral palsy
B Uncontrolled asthma
C Partial complex seizures
D Severe gastro-oesophageal reflux
E Immunodeficiency

3.66 A 12-year-old girl with a VSD presents with a week of fever, malaise and night sweats. When 2 years old she had a rash with Amoxil prescribed for otitis media. She has recently had a holiday in Brittany, but there are no known contacts with infection although her mother works in the local A&E. Examination reveals a temperature of 39°C, a grade 3 pansystolic murmur and some non-blanching erythematous maculopapular lesions on her arms and legs. The most relevant investigation is:

A Resting ECG
B Serum ASOT
C Urgent echocardiogram
D Chest radiograph
E Repeated blood cultures

3.67 **A parent comes to you for advice after her child's grommet insertion. What is the most important thing to tell her?**

A Swimming in a chlorinated pool is permitted

B Swimming in the sea should be avoided

C There may be short-term hearing loss

D Aeroplane flights should be avoided

E Plugging the ears for baths and showers is advisable

3.68 **A 6-year-old girl presents with soiling and she has never been toilet trained. She regularly passes normal formed stools into her underclothes without seemingly being concerned. Her parents separated when she was 3 and the mother has a history of an eating disorder. The father has a history of a duodenal ulcer. Her bowel habit was erratic and has much improved with lactulose 5 mL twice daily. Her examination is normal except for a slightly distended abdomen. The management plan most likely to succeed is:**

A Increase her laxatives

B Refer to Social Services

C Liaise with her schoolteacher

D Switch off her favourite TV programme whenever she soils

E Refer to the Child and Adolescent Mental Health Services (CAMHS)

PAPER 4

MULTIPLE CHOICE QUESTIONS

4.1 With regard to a cleft palate:

- ○ A It may cause hearing loss
- ○ B All babies with cleft palate should be admitted to the special care baby unit (SCBU) for nasogastric feeding (NG) feeding
- ○ C It should be repaired at 3 months
- ○ D Speech develops normally in approximately 75% of children
- ○ E It is associated with maternal epilepsy

4.2 The prevalence of asthma increases with:

- ○ A Female sex
- ○ B Family history of eczema
- ○ C Forceps delivery
- ○ D Passive smoking during pregnancy
- ○ E Urban living

4.3 With regard to infantile spasms:

- ○ A They are also known as 'salaam attacks'
- ○ B They usually start after 9 months
- ○ C They characteristically involve 'drop attacks' secondary to brief myoclonus or atonia
- ○ D The electroencephalogram (EEG) characteristically shows hypsarrhythmia in approximately 66%
- ○ E First-line treatment involves prednisolone or adrenocorticotrophic hormone (ACTH)

questions

4.4 Cerebral palsy:

A Is a contraindication to the pertussis vaccine
B May be secondary to hypoglycaemia in the perinatal period
C Features include the lack of primitive reflexes
D May be associated with impaired hearing
E Feeding difficulties arise from hypotonia

4.5 Risk factors for physical abuse include:

A Having a stepfather
B Recent parental divorce
C Birth at 31 weeks' gestation
D Being a child aged between 4 and 8 years
E Having grandparents living nearby

4.6 With regard to pica:

A It is defined as 'eating of things that are not food'
B It is usually an isolated behaviour
C The 'mouthing' of objects seen at about 8 months is a good example
D It is associated with iron deficiency anaemia
E Pica that does not respond to disciplinary approaches may require referral to a community paediatrician

4.7 Concerning hyperkinetic syndrome (attention deficit disorder or ADD):

A There is a boy:girl ratio of 10:1
B It may be associated with lead poisoning
C It may be associated with food additives
D It has an incidence of 5–10% in the USA
E Behavioural therapy is the mainstay of treatment

4.8 With regard to salicylate poisoning:

○ A It can cause respiratory alkalosis
○ B It can cause metabolic acidosis
○ C It can cause hypoglycaemia
○ D The child may be discharged if the 4-hour serum salicylate level is 800 mg/L
○ E Treatment may involve vitamin K and fresh frozen plasma (FFP)

4.9 With regard to the Mantoux test:

○ A It traditionally involves an injection into the extensor surface of the left forearm
○ B It should ideally be read between 48 and 72 h
○ C A positive result occurs when the area of induration is > 5 mm
○ D A negative result excludes tuberculosis (TB) infection
○ E Induration > 15 mm requires further investigation and possible anti-tuberculous chemotherapy

4.10 In sickle cell anaemia:

○ A Approximately 10% of African–Caribbean individuals in the UK carry haemoglobin (Hb) S
○ B Heterozygotes show hypochromia, target cells, Howell–Jolly bodies and occasional sickle cells on their blood film
○ C An antenatal diagnosis can be made
○ D Homozygotes are at an increased risk of biliary colic
○ E Painful crises develop from about 6 months of age in homozygotes

4.11 Reye syndrome:

A Is acute encephalopathy with fatty degeneration of the liver, kidneys and pancreas

B Is associated with ibuprofen exposure in young children

C Usually presents before the age of 2 years

D Is commonly complicated by hypoglycaemia

E Alanine aminotransferase (ALT), aspartate aminotransferase (AST) and bilirubin are usually elevated

4.12 With regard to Fallot's tetralogy:

A It typically has a left-to-right shunt

B It typically has a pansystolic murmur

C Cyanotic spells may be prevented by treatment with β blockers

D It has the characteristic chest radiological appearance of an 'egg lying on its side'

E Fallot's tetralogy and transposition of the great arteries (TGA) are the two leading causes of cyanotic congenital heart disease

4.13 Features of a headache that would support the diagnosis of a simple migraine include:

A Being preceded by transient visual field defects and micropsia

B Papilloedema

C Strabismus

D Diplopia

E Nystagmus

4.14 With regard to Down's syndrome:

○ A It is associated with an increased incidence of duodenal atresia

○ B It is the single most common cause of severe learning difficulty

○ C It is associated with hypothyroidism

○ D Trisomy 21 has a recurrence risk of 10%

○ E It is associated with general hypertonia

4.15 With regard to haemophilia:

○ A Haemophilia B is an autosomal recessive disorder

○ B Children with haemophilia A must never be given aspirin

○ C The prothrombin time is normal in both haemophilia A and haemophilia B

○ D Regular dental care is essential

○ E It is associated with progressive joint destruction

4.16 In chronic diarrhoea:

○ A Cows' milk protein intolerance is the most common cause in infants aged under 1 year in the UK

○ B Recognisable food in the stool suggests toddler diarrhoea

○ C Flat mucosa devoid of villa on a jejunal biopsy is diagnostic of coeliac disease

○ D Coeliac disease most commonly presents between 6 and 9 months of age

○ E Ulcerative colitis is inherited in an autosomal recessive manner

4.17 With regard to appendicitis:

○ A It is rare in the under-5s (< 2%)

○ B In the under-5s, nearly 90% of cases present with perforation

○ C Abdominal pain usually presents in the right iliac fossa

○ D Its differential diagnosis includes mesenteric adenitis, urinary tract infection (UTI) and diabetic ketoacidosis

○ E Assessing the child's ability to 'hop' helps exclude the diagnosis

4.18 The role of the health visitor includes:

○ A Supervising the running of immunisation clinics

○ B Reviewing the case notes of every child under 5 years who has attended A&E

○ C Child health surveillance in all children aged under 10 years

○ D Taking over postnatal care from the midwife at age 3 weeks

○ E Responsibility for supervision of children in care

4.19 With regard to anorexia nervosa:

○ A It affects 1 in 250 girls aged between 15 and 18 years

○ B Primary amenorrhoea may be present

○ C It is associated with hyperkalaemia

○ D It has a mortality rate of 1%

○ E It is characterised by having a disturbed perception of body image

4.20 Ophthalmology:

○ A Ophthalmia neonatorum is most commonly caused by *Neisseria gonorrhoeae*

○ B Stevens–Johnson syndrome is associated with iritis

○ C Orbital cellulitis is commonly secondary to adjacent sinusitis

○ D Glaucoma may be associated with aniridia

○ E Intrauterine toxoplasmosis infection results in an increased incidence of cataracts

4.21 With regard to adoption:

○ A The adopted child takes on the nationality of the adoptive parents

○ B Applicants must be aged 18 or over

○ C The natural parents must give their informed consent before the adoption can proceed

○ D The child must live with the adoptive parents for 6 months before the order is finalised

○ E At age 16 an adopted child is entitled to their original birth certificate

4.22 With regard to rickets:

○ A It is associated with seizures

○ B It may be secondary to ulcerative colitis

○ C It causes both genu valgum and genu varum

○ D Vitamin D-resistant rickets is an autosomal dominant condition

○ E It is associated with swelling at the wrists and costochondral junctions

questions

questions

4.23 Causes of generalised lymphadenopathy include:

○　A　Sarcoidosis
○　B　Kawasaki's disease
○　C　Phenytoin therapy
○　D　Eczema herpeticum
○　E　Juvenile chronic arthritis

4.24 Poor prognostic features of acute lymphoblastic leukaemia (ALL) include:

○　A　Age < 2 years
○　B　Age > 10 years
○　C　Being white
○　D　Male sex
○　E　Presenting white cell count (WCC) > 20 000/mm^3

4.25 With regard to inflammatory bowel disease:

○　A　Both Crohn's disease and ulcerative colitis are associated with finger clubbing, anaemia, erythema nodosum and arthritis
○　B　Crohn's disease has increased over the past 20–30 years and now affects about 5 per 10 000 individuals
○　C　Ulcerative colitis is characterised by inflammation of the whole thickness of the bowel wall, especially the terminal ileum and proximal colon
○　D　The 'string sign', 'skip lesions' and 'rose thorn ulcers' are characteristically seen in Crohn's disease after a barium meal and follow-through
○　E　Surgery is always required in the management of ulcerative colitis

4.26 Precocious puberty:

- ○ A Is defined as the onset of sexual maturation before 10 years of age in a girl
- ○ B Is associated with McCune–Albright syndrome
- ○ C Results in an increased final height
- ○ D Is commonly associated with intracranial tumours in boys
- ○ E Is associated with coeliac disease

4.27 With regard to bow legs (genu varum):

- ○ A They are normal in infants and usually correct by 5 years of age
- ○ B They may be secondary to osteogenesis imperfecta
- ○ C When caused by 'medial tibial torsion', they are associated with bowing of the tibia, which usually requires surgical correction
- ○ D They may be secondary to poliomyelitis
- ○ E They may be secondary to Osgood–Schlatter disease

4.28 A normal 18-month-old infant:

- ○ A Can balance on one foot for a second
- ○ B Can kick a ball forward
- ○ C Can walk upstairs holding on, one foot per step
- ○ D Can walk backwards
- ○ E May not be walking if a 'bottom shuffler'

4.29 With regard to HIV infection:

- ○ A The risk of vertical transmission in Europe is approximately 50%
- ○ B Breast-feeding should be avoided in developed countries
- ○ C It is a notifiable disease
- ○ D Pneumovax is contraindicated
- ○ E Testing for HIV antibodies helps to exclude neonatal congenital infection

4.30 A normal 3-year-old child:

- A Can lace up his or her own shoes
- B Will play interactive games (eg tag) with other children
- C Is not yet capable of imaginary play
- D Is 'dry' by day, but seldom at night
- E Is able to dress him- or herself without supervision

4.31 Most 3-year-old children:

- A Can recognise three colours
- B Will use more than 200 words but have greater comprehension
- C Can give first and last name
- D Can give definitions of more than 20 words
- E Comprehend the meaning of cold/tired/hungry

4.32 Inguinal hernia in infants:

- A Rarely requires surgical repair
- B Generally presents with strangulation
- C Should be repaired before 1 year of age
- D A significant proportion of inguinal hernias becomes irreducible before age 3 months
- E May contain an ovary

4.33 Mesenteric adenitis:

- A Often precedes an upper respiratory tract infection (URTI)
- B May give signs of peritonitis
- C Is caused by an adenovirus
- D Is not typically associated with a fever
- E Is associated with a lymphocytosis

4.34 The following associations are correct:

○ A Noonan syndrome and hypertrophic cardiomyopathy
○ B Turner's syndrome and a narrow carrying angle
○ C Edward syndrome and rocker bottom feet
○ D Pierre Robin syndrome and macrognathia
○ E Laurence–Moon–Biedl syndrome and night blindness

4.35 Language delay:

○ A When severe, has an incidence of approximately 1 in 5000
○ B Has an increased incidence among boys
○ C Is associated with cleft palate
○ D Reynell's Developmental Language Scale accurately assesses comprehension and expression
○ E Has an increased incidence in large families

EXTENDED MATCHING QUESTIONS

4.36 Theme: essential nutrients

○ A Calcium
○ B Folic acid
○ C Iron
○ D Vitamin A
○ E Vitamin B_6
○ F Vitamin B_{12}
○ G Vitamin C
○ H Vitamin D
○ I Vitamin E
○ J Zinc

For each of the cases, below please choose the nutritional element most likely to be deficient from the above list (each item may be used once or not at all):

1   A 6-year-old boy with cystic fibrosis is thought to have poor compliance with his medicines. He is failing to thrive and has mild ataxia and weakness.
2   A 4-year-old's parents are strict vegans. He is given iron supplements but is noted to be pale. His Hb is 9.2 g/dL.
3   A 2-year-old child is still exclusively breast-fed and has not yet started walking. He has prominent wrists and lumps round his sternum.

questions

4.37 Theme: respiratory conditions

- ○ A α_1-Anti-trypsin
- ○ B Atopic asthma
- ○ C Cystic fibrosis
- ○ D Foreign body inhalation
- ○ E Kartagener syndrome
- ○ F *Mycoplasma* infection
- ○ G Pertussis
- ○ H Recurrent aspiration
- ○ I Vascular ring
- ○ J TB

For each of the following cases, please choose the most likely diagnosis from the above list (each item may be used once or not at all):

1. A 2-year-old is referred with difficulty in breathing. She is noted to be wheezy – more on the right than the left. A chest radiograph reveals right-sided hyperexpansion.
2. An 18-month-old infant of a travelling family presents with an acute respiratory illness. Investigations at the time show a marked lymphocytosis. He has a persistent cough 2 months later.
3. A 3-year-old child has a recurrent nocturnal cough. He had mild eczema as an infant. He is otherwise well.

4.38 Theme: gastrointestinal disorders

- ○ A Abetalipoproteinaemia
- ○ B Coeliac disease
- ○ C Constipation with overflow
- ○ D Crohn's disease
- ○ E Giardiasis
- ○ F Ileal tuberculosis
- ○ G Lactose intolerance
- ○ H Toddler's diarrhoea
- ○ I Ulcerative colitis
- ○ J Viral gastroenteritis

For each of the following cases, please choose the most likely cause of the diarrhoea from the above list (each item may be used once or not at all):

1   A 9-year-old boy presents with a 2-month history of weight loss, abdominal pain and intermittent diarrhoea. There is no blood in the stool. He has a mildly tender abdomen and some perianal skin tags. Investigations reveal: C-reactive protein (CRP) 45 mg/dL, erythrocyte sedimentation rate (ESR) 50 mm in first hour.

2   A 3-year-old girl has a 2-month history of loose stools. Her parents are very concerned. The stools often contain 'undigested food'. She is otherwise well and thriving.

3   An 8-month-old infant has had watery diarrhoea for 4 days. There has been no recent travel. Her 2-year-old sibling has recently had a similar illness, although less severe. She is drinking her normal formula milk well and is not dehydrated.

4.39 Theme: endocrine disorders

○ A Chronic corticosteroid therapy
○ B Cystic fibrosis
○ C Constitutional delay in growth and puberty
○ D Growth hormone deficiency
○ E Hypochondroplasia
○ F Hypothyroidism
○ G Psychosocial deprivation
○ H Rickets
○ I Small genetic height potential
○ J Turner's syndrome

For each of the following cases of poor growth, please choose the most likely cause from the above list (each item may be used once or not at all):

1 A 7-year-old girl comes to outpatients with her parents who are concerned that she is too short. She has previously been fit and well. Her height and weight are both on the 2nd centile. Parental heights are on the 2nd (mother) and 10th (father) centiles.

2 A 13-year-old boy is the shortest in his class. He has no pubic or axillary hair and his testicular volume is 8 mL. His bone age is delayed.

3 A 9-year-old girl has previously had a bone marrow transplantation (matched sibling donor) for ALL. She presents because her growth is not keeping up with that of her peers. She is falling behind academically. She is gaining weight and has constipation.

questions

4.40 Theme: neurodevelopmental and psychological disorders

○ A Anorexia nervosa
○ B Asperger syndrome
○ C Attention deficit hyperactivity disorder (ADHD)
○ D Autism
○ E Depression
○ F Factitious illness
○ G Psychosocial deprivation
○ H Post-traumatic stress disorder
○ I Rett syndrome
○ J Temper tantrums

For each of the following cases, please choose the most likely diagnosis from the above list (each item may be used once or not at all):

1   A 3-year-old boy is brought to you because his mother is concerned about his attention span. You note that he has very poor eye contact and poor verbal skills (having only a four-word vocabulary). His weight and height are appropriate for his age.

2   A 4-year-old girl is referred for speech and language therapy because she speaks very little. She has not had her MMR (measles, mumps, rubella) or pre-school booster. She appears withdrawn and shy but will play games if encouraged. Her weight is on the 2nd centile for her age (2 years ago it was on the 50th). Her dentition is poor.

3   An 11-year-old girl is confrontational at home and argues with her parents. She enjoys going out with her friends. Her school performance is falling and her concentration is poor. She has had thoughts of deliberate self-harm in the past and presents with some superficial lacerations to her left wrist. Taking a detailed history, you elicit that she had been sexually assaulted by a family friend 1 year ago.

4.41 Theme: special investigations

○   A   Angiography
○   B   Bone scan
○   C   Computed tomography (CT)
○   D   Echocardiogram
○   E   Electrocardiogram (ECG)
○   F   Electroencephalogram (EEG)
○   G   Magnetic resonance imaging (MRI)
○   H   Plain radiograph
○   I   Positron emission tomography (PET)
○   J   Ultrasonography

For each of the following clinical problems, please choose the most useful investigation from the above list (each item may be used once or not at all):

1   A 2-year-old boy is diagnosed with and treated for Kawasaki's disease. You are concerned about possible complications and wish to investigate this.

2   A 1-year-old infant falls from a chair and hits her head on the concrete floor. She has a brief (1 min) seizure 4 h later.

3   A 4-year-old child is febrile and limping, complaining of pain in her left leg. There is some cellulitis overlying her distal left tibia.

4.42 Theme: rashes

○ A   Milia
○ B   Miliaria
○ C   Erythema toxicum
○ D   Staphylococcal septic spots
○ E   Neonatal acne
○ F   Infantile acne
○ G   Seborrhoeic dermatitis
○ H   Infantile eczema
○ I   Mongolian spot
○ J   Follicular eczema

For each of the conditions described below, please select the diagnosis from the list above.

1   A 2-day-old baby is noted to have numerous very small white spots over her nose. They have apparently been present since birth

2   A 3-day-old baby has yellow pustules over his lower abdomen, in both groin creases and also in the right axilla.

3   A 4-month-old child who was previously well develops comedones and inflamed papules over the cheeks and chin.

questions

questions

4.43 Theme: healthcare roles

○ A   Child psychiatrist
○ B   Psychologist
○ C   Educational psychologist
○ D   Physiotherapist
○ E   Occupational therapist
○ F   Orthoptist
○ G   Orthotist
○ H   Speech and language therapist
○ I   Dietician
○ J   School nurse

For each of the cases below, select from the list above the member of the multidisciplinary team who is not currently involved and would have an important role to play in the child's care:

1   A 4-year-old boy is on the autistic spectrum. He has been assessed by a clinical psychologist and an educational psychologist.

2   A 3-year-old child has quadriplegic cerebral palsy. She is suffering from contractures in her Achilles' tendon. She has extensive input from her physiotherapist and dietician.

3   A 7-year-old girl has polyarticular juvenile idiopathic arthritis (JIA). She has frequent flare-ups. There is good involvement of her physiotherapist, educational psychologist and school nurse.

BEST OF FIVE QUESTIONS

4.44 A 13-year-boy with asthma has frequent admissions and school absence despite being on 500 µg twice daily of an inhaled steroid, a long-acting β agonist twice daily and an oral leukotriene antagonist once daily. Your next step to improve control is:

A   Request a twice daily peak flow recording diary

B   Ask him to stop smoking

C   Review his inhaler technique

D   Address issues of adherence to the management plan

E   Obtain a school report

4.45 A 2-year-old boy has a 1 year history of intermittent urticaria, lasting 1–3 days every 3–4 weeks, and less frequent swelling of hands and feet. Your next action is to:

A   Prescribe an appropriate dose/weight of piriton twice daily

B   Prescribe a low-potency topical corticosteroid as needed

C   Request a detailed food and symptom diary

D   Request a blood assay for C1 esterase inhibitor

E   Prescribe a trial of an egg, milk and wheat elimination diet

questions

4.46 A 5-year-old girl has had recurrent blackouts over the previous 6 months. These were brief, lasting less than a minute during which some twitching of her hands and feet was noted. The recovery was rapid. These occurred almost exclusively during the daytime without warning when she was active. In the family the mother had similar episodes until adolescence, and a maternal uncle died suddenly in his teens. Clinically and developmentally she was normal. EEG, electromyogram (EMG) and serum biochemistry were normal.

- A Generalised tonic–clonic epilepsy
- B Reflex anoxic seizures
- C Breathholding attacks
- D Long Q–T syndrome
- E Syncope

4.47 A 15-year-old, previously healthy girl has had recurrent abdominal pain and intermittent diarrhoea over the previous year. During these episodes she may pass four to eight very loose stools with mucus. Over the past few months she has also passed stools mixed with blood during the attacks. Although she has not lost weight, her weight decreased by crossing a centile. She has not had her menarche. The mother suffers from vitiligo. Clinical examination was unremarkable: Hb 12.1 g/L; normal differential count; ESR 38 mm; autoantibody screen negative. The next most relevant investigation is:

- A Barium enema
- B Colonoscopy
- C Radio-isotope study
- D Abdominal radiograph
- E Angiography

4.48 A 5-month-old baby girl of a 16-year-old mother was referred with a 5-day history of cough, fever, rapid breathing and excessive crying. Antenatally, the mother was involved in a car accident as a passenger with no major injuries. The baby was born by vaginal delivery at 36 weeks and needed active resuscitation with intermittent positive pressure ventilation (IPPV) and received antibiotics for 5 days. Subsequent progress was uneventful. Birth weight was 2.48 kg (50th centile). On admission, weight was 4.2 kg (9th centile), and she was irritable and cried when handled. The respiratory rate was 55/min with vesicular breath sounds and bilateral crepitations. Chest radiograph showed slight hyperinflation. Unexpectedly fracture of left second, fifth and sixth ribs with well-formed callus was visible. Urea and electrolytes (U&Es), creatinine, Ca^{2+}, P and alkaline phosphatase were normal. A further skeletal survey did not reveal any other fractures. The most important action is:

- A Obtain a nasopharyngeal aspirate
- B Contact the health visitor
- C Obtain a per nasal swab
- D Refer urgently to Social Services
- E Isolate in a side room

questions

4.49 A 6-year-old Albanian boy was referred from the orthopaedic clinic for evaluation of his gait. According to the parents, he is falling and injuring himself in the playground and he is finding it increasingly difficult to keep up with other children. His development is grossly normal. General health has remained satisfactory. Parents are consanguineous. On examination growth is normal. The muscle mass was generally reduced, with enlargement of his calves. Reflexes were generally reduced, as was power, and hand–eye coordination normal. He used Gower's manoeuvre in getting up from floor. Urine and plasma amino acids and CT of the brain were normal. The most likely diagnosis is:

   A Cerebral palsy
   B Myasthenia gravis
   C Becker's muscular dystrophy
   D Guillain–Barré syndrome
   E Duchenne muscular dystrophy

4.50 A 7-year-old girl was admitted with high fever and a painful cough productive of blood-stained sputum. The clinical picture was that of right lower lobe pneumonia that was confirmed radiologically. She had a similar episode 9 months previously while away on holiday and was hospitalised for 3 days. The radiological report indicated identical changes at that time. There was no contact history of TB and she has not had the BCG (Bacille Calmette–Guérin). She was commenced on a course of antibiotics. The next most useful step in her management is:

   A Bronchoscopy
   B Mantoux test
   C CT of the thorax
   D Clinical and radiological review at follow-up
   E Ventilation–perfusion scan

4.51 A 2-and-a-half-year-old white boy presented with failure to thrive, recurrent respiratory infections and intermittent diarrhoea every 4–6 weeks since early infancy. He has been a fussy feeder throughout. He has also had intermittent oral ulcers and recurrent ear discharge. Stools varied from loose to formed with no blood or mucus. Weight and height are on 2nd centile (both parents' heights are on the 9th centile). Investigations were: Hb 11.0 g/dL. WBC 5 × 10^9/L with neutrophils 4 × 10^9/L and lymphocytes 0.5 × 10^9/L. Serum ferritin was 20 µg/L, serum IgA < 0.1 g/L, IgG 1.8 g/L, IgM 4.8 g/L. Sweat test: Na$^+$ 40 mmol, Cl$^-$32 mmol. IgA anti-transglutaminase antibodies were negative. On the basis of above history and findings the most likely diagnosis is:

   A Toddler's diarrhoea

   B Immune deficiency

   C Coeliac disease

   D Cystic fibrosis

   E Lactose intolerance

4.52 Which of the following is the most important addition to routine screening for a child with Down's syndrome at 12 months of age?

   A Plotting height and weight on standard growth charts

   B Urine dipstick for glucose

   C Urine dipstick for protein

   D Thyroid function tests (TFTs)

   E Dental screening

questions

4.53 A 4-year-old boy with haemophilia A presents with a suddenly swollen painful right knee. There is no history of trauma. He is known to have moderate severity of disease. Which of the following management options is most appropriate?

○ A Platelet transfusion
○ B Intravenous bolus DDAVP (desmopressin)
○ C Vitamin K intravenously
○ D Elevation of the limb and strict bed rest
○ E Infusion of recombinant factor VIII

4.54 A 12-hour-old baby boy is found to be jaundiced. Despite intravenous fluids and phototherapy, the serum bilirubin continues to rise and an exchange transfusion is performed. Mother's blood group is AB+, baby's blood group is O+. The baby's brother also became jaundiced as a neonate, though he needed only phototherapy. Which of the following is the most likely underlying diagnosis?

○ A Dehydration
○ B ABO incompatibility
○ C Rhesus haemolytic disease of the newborn
○ D G6PDH deficiency
○ E Gilbert's disease

4.55 A mother brings her 11-month-old child to you concerned about his head shape – you diagnose positional plagiocephaly. There is no evidence of torticollis or a sternomastoid tumour. What is the most appropriate course of action?

○ A Reassure her that it is a benign condition and requires no treatment

○ B Advise her to place the child's toys on the side of the cot that the child turns away from

○ C Referral to neurosurgical team for assessment and intervention

○ D Referral for a moulding helmet

○ E Advise her to place the child on his front to sleep.

4.56 A 4-year-old girl presents to A&E with abdominal pain and vomiting. She has been unwell for 3 days. On examination she is clinically 10% dehydrated, her pulse is 130 beast/min, respiratory rate (RR) 40/min, temperature 37.4°C. What investigation is most likely to provide a diagnosis?

○ A Arterial blood gas
○ B CRP level
○ C Amylase
○ D Full blood count (FBC)
○ E Blood glucose

4.57 Which of the following treatments is most appropriate for an 18-month-old child with head lice?

○ A Topical malathion
○ B Head shaving
○ C Topical permethrin
○ D Topical carbaryl
○ E Wet combing

questions

4.58 A parent brings in her 2-month-old infant for her immunisations. She wishes to know why the schedule has changed and why this child will not receive oral polio like the older siblings. What is the most appropriate explanation?

    A The new vaccine is more effective

    B The new vaccine is more convenient

    C There was variability in the virulence of the live attenuated vaccine

    D There is a risk of excretion of live vaccine virus to vulnerable individuals

    E There were more cases of vaccine polio than wild polio

4.59 A 15-year-old girl is seen in the A&E resuscitation room and is unrousable. Her pulse is 70 beats/min, RR 15/min and O_2 saturation (sats) 95% in air; she receives basic airway management and subsequently wakes up 30 min later at which point she is confused and aggressive. What is the drug that she is most likely to have taken?

    A Cannabis

    B Ecstasy (MDMA)

    C Cocaine

    D GHB (γ-hydroxybutyrate)

    E 'Poppers' (amyl nitrate)

4.60 A 5-year-old child is diagnosed with a periorbital cellulitis. Which of the following clinical signs would make you most concerned?

    A Spiking fever

    B Loss of pupillary reflex in that eye

    C Conjunctivitis in that eye

    D Headache

    E Nasal discharge

4.61 Prebiotics are added to many infant formulae. Which of the following is an evidence-based reason for their use?

- A Reduced risk of atopic dermatitis
- B Reduced risk of constipation
- C Improved neural development
- D Less gastro-oesophageal reflux
- E Less gastroenteritis

4.62 A 4-year-old girl completed treatment for acute myeloid leukaemia (AML) 6 months ago. She recently had a coryzal illness. She is brought to A&E with difficulty in breathing. On general examination she is pale and sweaty, pulse 110 beats/min, RR 40/min, sats 91% in air. On respiratory examination she has good air entry and no recession, but diffuse crackles throughout the lung fields. Cardiovascular examination reveals normal heart sounds with a gallop rhythm and no murmur. The only other finding of note is a liver edge 2 cm palpable below the costal margin. Her FBC is normal. What investigation is most likely to give a diagnosis?

- A Blood film
- B Bone marrow aspirate
- C Chest radiograph
- D Echocardiogram
- E CRP

4.63 A 14-year-old child with moderate depression is undergoing psychological therapy and family therapy. The depression appears to be unresponsive. What would be the most appropriate medication to start?

- A Amitriptyline
- B Sertraline
- C Diazepam
- D Paroxetine
- E Fluoxetine

4.64 A 7-year-old child presents to A&E with a 2-week history of a scaly rash on the right parietal area of his scalp. Over the last 2 days a 5 cm fluctuant swelling had developed, with the skin overlying it becoming erythematous. There are palpable posterior auricular lymph nodes on the same side. What is the best course of action?

A Referral for surgical incision and drainage

B Discharge home with oral Augmentin (co-amoxiclav) and review in 48 h

C Admit for intravenous antibiotics

D Start oral griseofulvin and flucloxacillin and arrange dermatology review

E Perform needle aspiration for culture and await results before starting treatment.

4.65 A 3-year-old boy had two episodes of severe colicky abdominal pain within 5 days, passing heavily blood-stained urine on the second occasion. The urine gradually cleared over the next 48 h. There was no fever, oliguria or swelling of the limbs. In other respects he was well. He is well nourished, not anaemic and has a BP of 88/52 mmHg. His abdomen was soft with no masses palpable. Hb 11.5 g/dL, WBC/differential count normal, U&Es and creatinine within the normal range. Urinalysis shows red cells +++ with urinary protein ++. The next most relevant investigation is:

A 24-hour oxalate excretion

B CT of abdomen

C Ultrasonography of kidneys, lower ureters and the bladder

D Serum calcium level

E MAG-3 scan

4.66 A 6-year-old girl presented after her first seizure, which was a generalised tonic–clonic episode that lasted for about 5 min. There was no associated fever. There was a 9-month history of headaches that occurred once in about 3–4 weeks, which were quite severe and needed analgesics. These were usually diurnal and not accompanied by nausea or vomiting. In between she had been normal with no change in her moods or behaviour. There is a strong family history of migraine, with the mother and maternal grandmother being affected. Clinical examination was normal. The most relevant investigation in the evaluation of the patient is:

- A Fasting blood sugar
- B EEG
- C CT of the brain
- D MRI of the brain
- E Trial with pizotifen

4.67 A 4-year-old on treatment for epilepsy with carbamazepine was admitted with a history of multiple bruising. She had had a seizure the previous day and had knocked her head during the attack, and now she has a large bruise over the forehead, in addition to several over her arms, legs and back. She had recently recovered from a flu-like illness and has had a course of cefalexin. She was previously on the Child Protection Register because of neglect and a violent father. Clinically, she appeared well and not anaemic, with small shotty lymph nodes on both sides of the neck. Multiple bruises and fine petechiae were noted over the trunk and limbs. Hb 11.3 g/dL, WBC 8.0×10^9/L, normal differential count, platelets $< 10 \times 10^9$/L, elevated anti-platelet antibody PaIgG; bone marrow showed increased megakaryocytes. Based on the above information, the most likely cause of her bruising is:

A   Glandular fever
B   ALL
C   Idiopathic thrombocytopenic purpura (ITP)
D   Carbamazepine-induced bone marrow suppression
E   Physical abuse

4.68 A 4-year-old girl was referred because of both day and night wetting. She has never been completely dry. She uses the toilet but continues to have constantly wet underwear. There is no history of dysuria, increased frequency or urgency. There is a past history of temper tantrums that is now less marked. Growth and development are normal: weight and height 25th centile; BP 80/50 mmHg. Perineal examination revealed a mild vulvitis and a normal introitus but dribbling of urine was noted. Ultrasonography of the bladder shows no urine residue. Three mid-stream specimens (MSUs) are normal and FBC, U&Es and creatinine are normal. The most likely cause of her problem is:

- A Bladder instability
- B Primary enuresis
- C Vesicoureteric reflux (VUR)
- D Duplex kidney(s) with ectopic ureter
- E Behavioural problem

Multiple Choice Answers

1.1 A, E

Pyloric stenosis has an incidence of 4 per 1000 live births, with boys being affected more than girls in a ratio of 4:1. Approximately 15% of affected infants have a positive family history, mainly on the mother's side. Vomiting occurs after feeds and is projectile but not bile stained, because the obstruction is so high. Persistent vomiting leads to hyperchloraemic/hypokalaemic alkalosis needing fluid replacement with 0.9% (physiological or normal) saline plus added potassium.

Examination may reveal an olive-shaped abdominal mass during a test feed and ultrasonography is the investigation of choice. A contrast upper gastrointestinal (GI) study is also useful, although seldom required, and may be associated with an increased risk of aspiration. Treatment is surgical by Ramstedt's pyloromyotomy.

1.2 A, E

The features of nephrotic syndrome include proteinuria, hypo-albuminaemia, generalised oedema and hyperlipidaemia. The serum albumin should be < 25 g/L with proteinuria > 1 g/m^2 per 24 h.

Peak incidence is between 2 and 5 years of age with most being the result of 'minimal change glomerulonephritis'. This accounts for 70–80% of cases of primary nephrotic syndrome, which has an incidence of approximately 2 in 100 000 in the UK, with a male:female ratio of 2:1. Over 90% respond to steroid therapy.

Diffuse proliferative glomerulonephritis accounts for about 10% of cases of primary nephrotic syndrome (focal segmental 10%, membranous 2%). Other causes of nephrotic syndrome include congenital and secondary causes (eg collagen disorders, diabetes mellitus, toxins). Initial management involves hospital admission for assessment and initiation of treatment, which may include corticosteroids, antibiotics, fluid management and diuretics. A high-protein, no-salt diet is poorly tolerated and a normal balanced diet provides adequate proteins. Salt restriction is used only if there is progressive oedema.

1.3   D, E

Low-birthweight (LBW) babies are those weighing < 2500 g, whereas very-low-birthweight (VLBW) babies weigh < 1500 g. Together they account for about 1 in 15 infants born in the UK. An LBW infant may be small for gestational age (SGA), ie < 10th centile, premature, ie born before 37/40, or both.

SGA babies may reflect maternal factors, such as chronic illness (eg chronic renal failure [CRF]), hypertension, smoking, alcohol and undernutrition, which results in placental insufficiency and therefore intrauterine growth retardation (IUGR). Maternal diabetes typically results in large-for-date babies, but can also result in small-for-dates babies.

Problems include an increased incidence of congenital malformations, intrapartum asphyxia, hypoglycaemia, impaired thermoregulation, respiratory distress syndrome in pre-term infants and jaundice. Survival has improved over the years, with over 95% of infants born weighing 2000–2500 g surviving, and only about 8% of surviving infants suffering a major handicap (eg cerebral palsy).

1.4   C, E

The indications for tonsillectomy include recurrent febrile convulsions associated with attacks of follicular tonsillitis, over three attacks of bacterial tonsillitis in two consecutive years, and tonsils that are so grossly enlarged between infections that they meet in the midline, causing noisy breathing, stertor or sleep apnoea. Primary postoperative haemorrhage occurs within 24 h and is usually the result of inadequate haemostasis, whereas secondary haemorrhage occurs between 7 and 10 days and is commonly caused by infection. Purulent follicular exudate may occur in both bacterial and viral tonsillitis. Some authorities claim that bacterial infection requires at least 10 days of antimicrobial treatment, to prevent rheumatic fever, although there is little relevance to this in developed countries.

Adenoidectomy is a useful treatment for glue ear, because the adenoids may encroach on the nasopharyngeal orifice of the eustachian tube. It can be performed at the same time as grommet insertion and myringotomy.

1.5   All false

Seventy-five per cent of children with autism are male and it usually develops before 3 years of age. Typical features of autism include: global impairment of language and communication; impairment of social relationships, especially empathy; and ritualistic and compulsive phenomena. All three features should be present to make a diagnosis. The 'idiot savant' is a rare feature of autism; most children have a decreased IQ.

The treatment of autism includes: educational and behavioural modification programmes; and parental support and guidance. Drugs such as *tranquillisers are rarely used and only for severe behavioural difficulties resulting in self-harm*, whereas haloperidol may be used to reduce stereotypes (although use of haloperidol is decreasing). Finally, residential placement may be necessary in severe cases where families are unable to cope; indeed up to 60% of such individuals need long-term hospital or institutional care.

1.6   B, C, E

Vulvovaginitis is the most common gynaecological disorder in girls. Commonly isolated organisms in pre-pubertal girls include *Gardnerella* spp., *Bacteroides* spp. and streptococci. Threadworms may also cause symptoms and a vaginal foreign body should be considered if the discharge is bloodstained or offensive. Risk factors of infection include the lack of labial fat pads protecting the vaginal orifice and lack of the protective acid secretions found during the reproductive years.

Treatment includes: antibiotics if a specific organism is present; exclusion of an underlying cause, eg recent broad-spectrum antibiotics; attention to vulval hygiene and avoidance of irritants; and topical dienestrol cream in refractory cases, which is said to work *by improving the acidity*. If the symptoms are not persistent, and in the absence of any other physical or behavioural signs or psychosocial risk factors, the risk of sexual abuse is small and does not have to be discussed.

answers

127

answers

1.7 A, B, E

Routine blood pressure measurement in children is not part of a screening test but should be done routinely during the cardiovascular examination. In particular, if there are signs of malignant hypertension (eg papilloedema), renal or adrenal masses, renal artery bruit, goitre, radial–femoral delay and neurofibromatosis found on examination. The correct cuff size is approximately two-thirds the length of the upper arm. The fifth Korotkoff sound is often not heard in childhood, so the fourth is used until adolescence, when the fifth is used. In infants it is easier to use Doppler ultrasonography, or more typically an oscillatory method such as the Dinamapp. Results can be checked against normal values for age.

Secondary hypertension is more common in younger than in older children. After 13 years, 50% is caused by primary hypertension and 50% by secondary hypertension (of which 80% is the result of renal parenchymal disease, 10% renal vascular disease and 10% 'other'). The level of hypertension requiring treatment is not really known but most clinicians treat a diastolic blood pressure > 90 mmHg before 13 years and > 100 mmHg after 13 years. Note that three or so recordings should be taken some weeks apart (in general) before a diagnosis of hypertension is made.

1.8 B, E

If an infant suffers a cot death it is important to ensure the health of all siblings, especially the surviving twin, who is at increased risk and should always be admitted for observation, full septic screen and possible investigations for inherited metabolic disorders. Other risk factors include viral infections, hyperthermia (from over-wrapping/prone sleeping position), old PVC mattresses and parental smoking; indeed parents who stop smoking have been shown to decrease the risk of their child suffering a cot death significantly.

Apnoea monitors do not decrease the incidence of cot death and their use is controversial. Advantages include reassurance, ease of use and portability. However, they are expensive and often lead to false alarms and increased anxiety. All parents issued with an alarm must be trained in basic life support. Parents should be taught to recognise and assess signs of illness in their babies, and a system of increased surveillance by the health visitor and GP should be in place.

Parents should be encouraged to consult their GP more readily and should not be criticised for this.

1.9 B, D

More than 70% of acute bronchiolitis is the result of RSV; the rest is secondary to adenovirus, rhinovirus, parainfluenza 1, 2 and 3, and influenza A. The virus may be detected in a nasopharyngeal aspirate by immunofluorescence. Ribavirin is an antiviral agent of limited effectiveness against RSV and, as it is very expensive and difficult to administer, it is usually considered only for 'high-risk' babies (eg pre-term infants, bronchopulmonary dysplasia, congenital heart disease) and severely ill individuals. Salbutamol and theophylline have no effect on bronchiolitic obstruction in those aged under 1 year and there is limited evidence that ipratropium bromide is beneficial. Maternal IgG is protective against RSV.

1.10 A, D, E

Atopic eczema is very common, affecting up to 10% of children, and its incidence is increasing. It generally occurs before 6 months, but can start at any age. Of cases 50% have resolved by 5 years and 80% by 10 years. It may occur anywhere, but favours flexor surfaces in older children. Chinese herbal treatment has been shown to be effective, although its mechanism is unknown and adverse effects such as liver enzyme derangement are well documented. Initial treatment includes preventive measures such as avoidance of irritants and feeding high-risk infants with breast or hypoallergenic formula milks. Breast-feeding mothers may also consider avoiding consumption of common food allergens (eg cows' milk or eggs), although the evidence base for this is weak. Other more active treatment methods include skin emollients, topical steroids and antibiotics for secondary infection.

1.11 B, D, E

Truancy is associated with children aged over 8 years whereas school refusal commonly occurs in children aged between 5 and 11 years. School refusal occurs typically in a small, conventional social class I or II family who may collude over their child's non-attendance. The prevalence is similar in boys and girls (truancy being more common in boys) and it commonly presents with various psychosomatic features.

1.12 A, C, D, E

Causes of persistent snoring include hypertrophic nasal turbinates, allergic rhinitis, deviated nasal septum, nasal polyps, obesity and hypothyroidism. Recurrent tonsillitis may result in permanently enlarged tonsils, which predispose to persistent snoring, as do the macroglossia and other midfacial abnormalities associated with Down's syndrome.

1.13 A, B

Of infants with OA 85% will have a tracheo-oesophageal fistula and 30% will have another abnormality. OA may be part of the 'VACTERL' syndrome (ie vertebral, anorectal, cardiovascular, tracheo-oesophageal, renal and limb anomalies). Mothers typically have polyhydramnios antenatally.

It is diagnosed by the inability to pass a catheter into the stomach, which will be seen on a radiograph to be coiled in the oesophagus. Contrast radiography should be avoided because of the risk of aspiration. A tracheo-oesophageal fistula *without* an OA may present with recurrent pneumonia.

1.14 A, B, C, D

The stepping reflex persists from birth to 6–8 weeks only.

1.15 A, B

Treatment of cystic fibrosis includes regular (twice daily) chest physiotherapy and postural drainage, which is essential in preventing and treating chest infections – the parents usually do this. A small number of children have had successful heart and lung transplantations; however, availability of suitable donors is limited and for most chronic patients surgery is not an option because of their poor general condition. Prophylactic flucloxacillin or other anti-staphylococcal antibiotics are helpful in preventing staphylococcal chest infections, although there are conflicting opinions over the efficacy of this policy. Acute infections should be treated with 'best guess' antibiotics until cultures become available.

Patients have high-energy requirements and therefore need a high-calorie diet with normal protein and carbohydrate and high fat content. Fat restriction is no longer recommended because fat is the most energy-dense food. Supplemental pancreatic enzymes should be taken before all meals and snacks to prevent the clinical features of pancreatic insufficiency.

1.16   C, E

Screening tests should have a high sensitivity (ie few false negatives) and high specificity (ie few false positives). Screening tests should be inexpensive; however, calculation of the true cost should include the money saved by detection of the disease at an early stage, so 'cost-effective' is probably a more accurate term. The screening test should also be easy to perform, acceptable to the patient, repeatable and produce a yield of at least 1 in 10 000 positive diagnoses of a treatable condition. Effective screening tests are available for a limited number of conditions. Ideally the defined condition screened for should be an important one with a recognisable latent or early symptomatic stage and a well-known natural history if untreated. Screening must be a continuous process to be effective and not a 'one off'. Screening tests are ideally undertaken in primary care.

1.17   B, C, E

Migraines are generally preceded by an 'aura', which varies depending on which artery is affected. Vasoconstriction of a cranial artery may result in a transient oculomotor nerve palsy, ataxia, hemiparesis or aphasia. Intracranial pathology usually results in some permanent residual neurology. Migraine sufferers have a positive family history in 80% of cases, whereas acute severe headaches with no past medical or family history are more indicative of intracranial pathology. A significant space-occupying lesion may present with personality change, and headaches that wake the child at night and are worse in the morning. Headaches may occur daily, escalating in a crescendo pattern; they may be accompanied by vomiting and a stiff neck and are exacerbated by coughing and bending over. 'Exclusion diets' are of no benefit and are sometimes used in the management of migrainous headaches, which should also respond to other simple measures such as analgesics and antiemetics.

1.18 A, C

Soto syndrome (cerebral gigantism), Klinefelter syndrome and Marfan syndrome are all associated with tall stature.

1.19 A, B, D

Conditions that may result in a false-positive sweat test include Addison's disease, hypothyroidism, nephrogenic diabetes insipidus, glucose-6-phosphatase dehydrogenase (G6PDH) deficiency, mucopolysaccharidosis and ectodermal dysplasia. Bronchiectasis is a clinical feature of cystic fibrosis, but will not cause a positive sweat test as such.

1.20 A, D, E

Part III of the Education Act 1993 is the legislation in the UK dealing with special educational needs (it replaces the Education Act 1981). Its emphasis is on the earliest possible identification of SEN, including pre-school children, and the importance of partnership of parents, children, schools, local education authorities (LEAs) and any other involved agencies. It aims to teach a wide and balanced curriculum, including the National Curriculum, and most children with SEN, including those with Statements, will have their needs met in mainstream schools.

Statements of SEN should be made and reviewed annually.

A child has a learning difficulty if he or she has a significantly greater difficulty in learning than most children of the same age or has a disability that either prevents or hinders the child from making use of the educational facilities provided for children of the same age in schools within the LEA's area. Special educational provision includes any educational provision that is additional to or different from that provided by mainstream schools for a child aged over 2 years or any educational provision given to a child aged under 2 years.

1.21 A, D

Accidents are the single largest cause of death in children aged between 1 and 14 years and are responsible for approximately a third of all childhood deaths. Falls are the most common accident; however, road accidents (< 5% of all accidents) are the most common fatal accident, accounting for about 50% of accidental deaths. Approximately 15% of all children per year attend A&E because of an accidental injury; most of these are boys aged 5–8 years from social classes IV and V.

1.22 A, C, D, E

Bilirubin toxicity is caused by free unconjugated bilirubin that is lipid soluble and therefore readily crosses brain cell membranes. Kernicterus is rare in term infants if the serum bilirubin does not exceed 380 mmol/L; however, pre-term infants or those with sepsis, hypoxia or acidosis may be affected at much lower levels. Symptoms include poor feeding, irritability, hypertonicity or hypotonicity, opisthotonus, high-pitched cry, apnoea and convulsions.

Treatment involves phototherapy using narrow-spectrum blue light of wavelength 450–475 nm, which causes photo-isomerisation and photo-oxidation of bilirubin to less lipophilic pigments. Management should also include ensuring adequate hydration and possible exchange transfusion. If the baby survives, long-term sequelae include choreoathetoid cerebral palsy, high-frequency nerve deafness, paralysis of upward gaze and developmental delay.

1.23 A, B, C, D, E

All are safe to use during breast-feeding; however, thyroxine may interfere with neonatal screening for hypothyroidism.

1.24 A, B, C, D, E

Nose picking is the most common cause of epistaxis in children, which is usually from the blood vessels on the nasal septum (Little's area). Other common causes include upper respiratory tract infections (URTIs), allergic rhinitis and foreign bodies. Rarer causes include bleeding disorders and tumours of the nose and sinuses. Hypertension is a common cause of epistaxis in adults, but is rare in children.

1.25 C, D, E

There are 20 deciduous or 'milk' teeth and 32 permanent teeth (including four wisdom teeth). Teething may cause irritability, excessive salivation and a flushed appearance, but there is no fever. The first tooth to appear is generally a lower central incisor. Most children do not have the hand–eye coordination (or attention span) to clean their teeth adequately until about 8–10 years of age, so parents should re-brush their children's teeth at least once a day. Adequate cleaning is enough to clear the pits of the deciduous molars, clear the gum line of plaque and supply effective fluoride application – this requires a high level of fine motor skill and is recommended in adults to last at least 2 min (30 s per quadrant) – much longer than it sounds, and not easy even for adults to do correctly. Thumb sucking may result in malocclusion and requires an orthodontic assessment.

1.26 A, C

Infants with a urinary tract infection (UTI) may present with vomiting, irritability and feeding problems. Between 2 and 5 years abdominal pain, fever, dysuria and frequency are classic, whereas schoolchildren have the more adult picture of dysuria, frequency, haematuria and loin pain, commonly without fever. Vesicoureteric reflux is found in approximately 35% of younger children with a UTI. There is said to be a significant risk of progressive renal damage in the under-2s; thus prompt diagnosis and treatment is essential in children aged under 2, who should be investigated during or after their first UTI. Bacteria multiply rapidly at room temperature and should be 'plated' within 1 h of collection. However, if this is not possible they may be refrigerated for up to 24 h. Pyuria occurs in 50% of UTIs; however, there are other causes of pyuria including fever from other causes, trauma, some drugs (eg diuretics), calculi and renal TB.

1.27 A, D

Scabies is caused by the *Sarcoptes scabiei* mite, which burrows into the skin to lay eggs. Typical sites include the interdigital webs and flexor aspects of the wrists of older children and adults; however, in infants the face and scalp are often involved as well. *Sarcoptes scabiei* is transmitted by close contact and has an incubation period of 2–4 weeks. Therefore, the whole family must be treated with γ-benzene hexachloride lotion on two occasions, 7 days apart to ensure eradication. Clothing and bedding should be decontaminated by hot washing.

Pruritus, which is usually worse at night, is a result of sensitisation and persists for 4–6 weeks after eradication. Symptomatic measures such as calamine lotion or antihistamine should be tried and further re-treatment avoided because this will lead to irritant dermatitis and resistance.

1.28 A, B, C, D

Orthopaedic complications of obesity include Blount's disease and slipped femoral epiphyses. Most obese healthy children are tall for their age with advanced bone age. If an obese child is short for age it is important to exclude hypothyroidism, growth hormone deficiency, Cushing's disease, and Down's and Prader–Willi syndromes.

1.29 A, D, E

The ketogenic diet is beneficial in some children with intractable seizures; however, it is unpalatable and difficult to enforce. Protective helmets should be worn while cycling; however, cycling (like swimming) must be supervised and busy/open roads avoided. It is also important that restrictions are kept to a minimum and education in mainstream schools should be the goal, with teachers kept informed about progress and drug treatment. Neurosurgery is indicated in a few, carefully selected children with refractory epilepsy.

1.30 A, B, D, E

Hirschsprung's disease presents with constipation. It is caused by a congenital absence of intestinal autonomic ganglion cells of the Auerbach and Messier plexus, and is also associated with hypertrophy of extrinsic autonomic nerves. Causes of constipation include a low-fibre diet, over-enthusiastic potty training, anal trauma (eg postoperative, abuse), medication, dehydration, hypercalcaemia, hypothyroidism and spinal disorders (eg spina bifida). Anal fissures exacerbate pre-existing constipation and can be caused by constipation but, very rarely, actually cause constipation in themselves.

1.31 B, C, D, E

Phenylketonuria is an autosomal recessive condition with an incidence of 1:7000 in the UK. A heel-prick blood test (the so-called Guthrie test) at day 6 includes a screening test for PKU (elevated levels of phenylalanine) and for congenital hypothyroidism. PKU is associated with infantile spasms and will result in mental disability if the diagnosis is delayed and dietary restrictions not enforced. These restrictions should be continued until the child is at least 10 years old and ideally until adulthood. However, dietary restrictions should always be reinstated before conception and maintained throughout pregnancy to improve outcome, because genetically normal babies may be affected antenatally by the elevated levels of phenylalanine in the maternal circulation.

1.32 B, C, D, E

1.33 A, B

Acute lymphoblastic leukaemia is the leading paediatric malignancy and accounts for 85% of all childhood leukaemias. The peak incidence is between 2 and 6 years, with boys being slightly more affected than girls (55% versus 45%). Common presenting features include sepsis, lethargy, pallor, bleeding, bruising, petechiae, skeletal pain secondary to leukaemic infiltration, lymphadenopathy and hepatosplenomegaly. Investigations include a blood film that reveals anaemia, thrombocytopenia and usually circulating blast cells and a bone marrow aspiration. ALL is subdivided according to its immunological surface membrane markers, with 'common' having the best prognosis and 'B cell' the worst. Treatment involves ensuring good hydration, and allopurinol before chemotherapy in order to avoid renal impairment from urate stone formation. Epstein–Barr virus is associated with an increased incidence of Burkitt's lymphoma.

1.34 A, B, D

Spina bifida occulta is seen in 5–10% of all children and is usually found incidentally on a radiograph. In a meningocele, the dorsal laminae are absent with a skin-covered lesion containing only cerebrospinal fluid (CSF) with no underlying neurological involvement. Myelomeningocele is associated with neurological involvement. The neurological deficit depends on the level of the lesion, but double incontinence is the norm with paraplegia of the lower limbs. Both spastic and flaccid paralyses are seen, but the latter is more typical. In 90% of affected children hydrocephalus develops, which is most commonly secondary to an Arnold–Chiari malformation.

1.35 B, D

The characteristic incubation periods for the following conditions are: chickenpox (10–24 days); measles (7–14 days); glandular fever (30–50 days); mumps (12–31 days); and rubella (14–21 days).

answers

Answers to Extended Matching Questions

1.36 Analysis of blood gases

Table 1 Normal ranges

	Normal range
pH	7.35–7.45
P_{CO_2}	4.5–5.5 kPa
P_{O_2}	6.5–13.5 kPa
HCO_3^-	25–35 mmol/L
BE (Base excess)	−1 to +1 mmol/L

Capillary samples: approximate normal ranges are as given in Table 1.

However, Pa_{CO_2} upper limits can be allowed up to 6.5 kPa. Lower Pa_{CO_2} values can be permitted on venous samples; however, if oxygenation is the concern, an arterial sample should be taken (capillary samples are well arterialised and can be interpreted as arterial).

1   B – Compensated respiratory acidosis

The Pa_{CO_2} is raised, but the pH is normal so this is a fully compensated gas. Given the history, this is a compensated respiratory acidosis.

2   G – Partially compensated metabolic acidosis

A pH of 7.32 is mildly acidotic, so the likely diagnosis is diabetic ketoacidosis. The HCO_3^- is low so this is a metabolic acidosis; however, the Pa_{CO_2} is low (2.9 kPa) so there is some respiratory compensation (though NOT fully).

3   D – Metabolic alkalosis

An alkalotic gas: the Pa_{CO_2} is slightly raised and there is a very raised HCO_3^-; this is consistent with a metabolic alkalosis. (The likely diagnosis in this child is pyloric stenosis or possibly a pre-ampullary duodenal stenosis – leading to loss of H^+ and Cl^- in the vomit.)

1.37 Immunisations

1   J – HIV-infected children should not receive BCG
Some experts advise that measles vaccine can be given if the child has a CD4 count > 200. Mumps and rubella vaccines can be given singly.

2   C – Normal immunisation schedule
Autism is not a contraindication to any immunisation.

3   C – Normal immunisation schedule
Children with sickle cell trait should receive the universal schedule. Those with sickle cell disease should receive the unconjugated vaccine at age 2–3 years, in addition to the conjugated vaccine as part of the universal schedule (Table 2).

Table 2 Current immunisation schedule (as of November 2006)

Age	Immunisation
2 months	DTaP/Hib/IPV + PCV
3 months	DTaP/Hib/IPV + MenC
4 months	DTaP/Hib/IPV + MenC + PCV
12 months	Hib + MenC
13–15 months	MMR + PCV
3½–5 years	MMR + DTaP/IPV
13–18 years	dT + IPV

Key: DTaP/Hib/IPV, diphtheria, tetanus, acellular pertussis/ *Haemophilus influenzae* b/inactivated polio vaccine (available as '5 in 1' or pentavalent vaccine); PCV, pneumococcal conjugate vaccine; MenC, meningitis C; MMR, measles, mumps and rubella; dT, 'low-strength' diphtheria toxoid + tetanus.

Note that BCG is NOT part of the UK's universal schedule but may be offered in areas of high TB incidence.

answers

1.38 Infant milk formulae

1   E – High-energy formula

The chronic lung disease means that the infant uses more calories to breathe and therefore has a higher than normal daily calorie requirement. A higher calorie formula is needed and a high-energy formula would be most appropriate. Pre-term formulae are more calorific but unsuitable for infants of this age.

2   A – Breast milk

In the UK, maternal HIV, current cytotoxic therapy or galactosaemia in the infant is the only medical reason not to breast-feed.

3   F – Hydrolysed protein formula

The clinical scenario fits with a cows' milk protein intolerance. Gastro-oesophageal reflux is associated with cows' milk protein intolerance as a result of eosinophil infiltration in the oesophagus. Soya formulae are not recommended for infants aged under 6 months because they contain phyto-oestrogens.

1.39 Epilepsy

1 J – Rolandic epilepsy

These features best fit with 'benign' rolandic epilepsy. The age of onset and type of seizure are typical. The centrotemporal spikes are diagnostic. The term 'benign' rolandic epilepsy is slightly misleading in that, although the outcome is usually good with the seizures disappearing by adulthood, the nocturnal seizures are increasingly linked to SUDEP (sudden unexplained death in epilepsy). The risk of SUDEP lowers the threshold of many clinicians to start antiepileptics.

2 A – Absence epilepsy

Absence seizures are often first noticed as 'poor concentration' at school. The child is concentrating but is having absences that may be mistaken for daydreaming. Classically, 3/s spikes on EEG are seen. In an outpatient setting hyperventilation is a useful stimulus to bring on a seizure, thus making the diagnosis.

3 B – Complex partial seizures (of the temporal lobe)

The prodromal features described, and the type of seizure described, are common in temporal lobe epilepsy.

1.40 Rashes

1   F – Pityriasis rosea

The presence of the single spot and then the development of this rash fit very well with the 'Herald' patch and 'Christmas tree' rash of pityriasis rosea. Pityriasis is probably viral in origin but the exact causative organism is unknown. The rash appears 1–2 weeks after the Herald patch, lasts 2 weeks and then slowly resolves. Treatment is symptomatic.

2   A – Erysipelas

Slapped-cheek syndrome is possible but this child is systemically unwell and the cheeks are cellulitic. Erysipelas is commonly caused by group A streptococci. Treatment is with intravenous penicillin.

3   G – Rubella

Rubella has an incubation period of 2–3 weeks. The rash appears on the face, spreads down to the trunk and then finally affects the limbs. Cervical, occipital and posterior auricular lymph nodes are often enlarged before the appearance of the rash.

1.41 Renal diseases

1   G – Post-streptococcal glomerulonephritis

Red urine probably indicates haematuria. He is hypertensive and is having symptomatic headaches; these two features fit with a nephritis. A low C3 and normal C4 count are typical for post-streptococcal glomerular nephritis.

2   E – Mesangial IgA nephropathy

Although he has had a recent URTI, the onset of the symptoms is too soon after the URTI for post-streptococcal glomerular nephritis (which is normally more than a week after). In addition his blood pressure is normal (which doesn't fit with a nephritis), and the complement levels are normal.

3   C – Haemolytic uraemic syndrome

Any renal impairment following a diarrhoeal episode should raise the suspicion of HUS. This is confirmed by a very high urea, low Hb and low platelets. Examination of a blood film would show a microangiopathic haemolytic anaemia. HUS is the most ommon cause of acute renal failure in childhood. It is caused by verotoxins produced by *Escherichia coli* 0157 (a cause of bloody diarrhoea). Over half of the cases require dialysis.

1.42 The unwell infant

1   A – Cardiac failure

Difficulty completing feeds, along with sweating, is a good indicator of heart failure in infancy. Hepatomegaly is another sign of cardiac failure. It is important to distinguish between cardiac failure (not cyanotic and caused by a right-to-left shunt), and duct-dependent cardiac lesions (duct dependent: so when duct, closes infant becomes cyanotic).

2   F – Galactosaemia

The features of hepatomegaly, jaundice and abnormal clotting go together with both sepsis and hepatitis caused by galactosaemia. The urine-reducing sugars would be negative in sepsis – although in these cases in practice you would treat for sepsis as well.

3   I – Non-accidental injury (NAI)

NAI, HDN (haemorrhagic disease of the newborn) and group B streptococcal sepsis are the three main possibilities in this case. HDN is less likely because the baby is bottle-fed and should therefore be getting sufficient vitamin K. If this were HDN, it would probably be an acute event, and the fact that the baby is 'always' crying points against this and more towards NAI.

answers

1.43 Immunodeficiency

1   A – IgA deficiency

IgA has an incidence of approximately 1 in 500. Recurrent upper and lower respiratory infections are the most common symptoms. Recurrent otitis media is often reported. There is an association with atopic and autoimmune conditions. Treatment is with antibiotics for acute infections and consideration of prophylactic antibiotics.

2   B – SCID

Children with severe combined immunodeficiency (SCID) are often well for the first couple of months. The usual presentation is at 3–4 months with recurrent/persistent diarrhoea and growth faltering. Candidiasis is often present. Other presentations include atypical infections and infections (especially chest) that are difficult to treat.

3   E – HIV infection

The risk of vertical transmission of HIV in Europe is 10–25%. The risk is minimised by anti-retroviral agents and delivery by caesarean section. Presentation in infancy is often with failure to thrive. Gastrointestinal symptoms are common. Serum immunoglobulins may show a hyper-IgG globinaemia with a low IgM/IgA. Diagnosis is on HIV PCR (polymerase chain reaction) and p24 antigen detection (HIV antibodies may be present as a result of maternal infection and placental passage).

Best of Five Answers

1.44 D

Although Down's, Prader–Willi and Beckwith–Wiedemann syndromes can all present with neonatal hypotonia, they are not severe enough to cause respiratory insufficiency.

1.45 C

The most important step to take is to check inhaler technique before going to the next stage of the British Thoracic Society (BTS) guidelines. If the current medication is not being effectively given, there is no point in increasing the medication.

1.46 E

These are the clinical features of bronchiolitis – most frequently caused by RSV, but also by adenovirus and influenza virus. These features do not really fit with croup. Virally induced atopic wheeze is possible.

1.47 D

If the parents are unmarried then the father has no legal parental responsibility. Although the law was changed in 2004 to give parental rights to non-married fathers who appear on the birth certificate, this will not apply retrospectively – ie if a child is born before December 2004 the father has no parental responsibility if not married to the mother.

Therefore, only the mother can consent to procedures on the child. The child can consent for him- or herself once 'competent' (see Gillick competence on page 207 (answer to 3.50)). It is very unlikely that a 10-year-old child would be competent to consent to an operation (appreciating the risks of anaesthesia). An important point is that, even if a child can consent to a procedure when competent (if under 16), legally he or she cannot refuse one if the person with parental responsibility consents.

1.48 B

Breast development is the first sign of puberty in girls (from 8 years). Menarche occurs approximately 2 years later (at Tanner stage 4). Peak height velocity will usually coincide with menarche. There is a wide range in the times of onset of the stages.

(A good reference for the sequence of development is: Marshall WA, Tanner JM 1969. Variations in pattern of pubertal changes in girls. *Archives of Diseases in Childhood* 44:291–303.)

1.49 A

As this child is afebrile, septic arthritis and irritable hip are unlikely. Irritable hip is uncommon in this age group anyway (usually affecting those aged 1–4 years). Osgood–Schlatter disease is pain caused by inflammation of the patellar tendon at the tibial insertion. Slipped upper femoral epiphysis occurs classically in adolescence (M:F = 3:2).

1.50 D

This is the best interpretation of clinical governance. The other statements are all important 'pillars' (parts) of clinical governance but none individually encapsulates the whole concept.

1.51 D

This is the only explanation that fits. In poor compliance TSH rises as T_4 is repeatedly missed; however, when the child has to come for TFTs, T_4 is restarted and so the plasma T_4 rapidly reverts to normal, although TSH is slower to recover.

1.52 B

Food intolerance is a difficult area, with parents wanting definitive tests and answers. The only scientific and practical way of 'detecting' intolerance is to remove the suspected foodstuff and see if there is an improvement in symptoms. A staggered reintroduction of individual foods can then be tried to see if the symptoms recur. RAST and skin-prick tests have some limitations in both specificity and sensitivity, and need to be interpreted in combination with the clinical history. A well, thriving child is less likely to have serious pathology (although you should always keep this in the back of your mind).

1.53 D

External angular dermoid is by far the most likely diagnosis. External angular dermoids (dermoid cysts) are embryological remnants that contain dermal and epidermal tissues. The site of the lump means that the other options are much less likely. Neurofibromas are uncommon in children this young.

1.54 B

Neurodevelopment is a dynamic process. Infants achieve 'milestones' gradually; as an example they do not suddenly sit unsupported one morning, having been unable to the previous morning. There is an inherent variation in when a child will achieve a 'milestone', and it is important to know the range of ages at which it is normal to develop skills. The Denver II chart is a useful tool, which shows the normal progression of development and the ranges at which certain milestones occur. If a child has not achieved a milestone by the age at which 90% of the population would be expected to have achieved it, then further assessment may be indicated.

If a child is delayed in one of the neurodevelopmental areas, that may well affect the development of another area:

- Sitting unsupported: by 8 months

- Pull to stand: by 10 months

- Rolling prone to supine: by 7 months (supine to prone 1 month later)

- Climb up stairs without support: by 20 months

- Transferring hand to hand (actually a fine motor milestone!): by 7 months

NOTES ON DEVELOPMENTAL ASSESSMENT

answers

Development is the maturation of the nervous system and is dependent on experience/stimulus. By the end of the second trimester, the fetal brain has a full complement of nerve cells; however, neurodevelopment is the maturation of these cells and the development of connections between them.

Development depends on the stimulation to develop and, importantly, loss of primitive reflexes and development of acquired reflexes.

Remember the Areas of Development

- Gross motor
- Fine motor and vision
- Speech and hearing
- Social.

Gross motor

The gross motor skills develop in a 'cephalo-caudal' manner (from the head working downwards). This means that head control is one of the earliest gross motor milestones achieved and is usually followed by lifting of the shoulder when prone, and gradually getting better truncal control, sitting up, crawling then walking. Gross motor skills are very dependent on the loss of primitive reflexes and development of acquired reflexes. An infant will not be able to sit unsupported if the lateral saving reflex (putting arms out laterally to stop falling sideways) hasn't developed. Likewise if the parachute reflex (putting arms out in front to stop falling forwards) does not develop then a child will not be able to learn to walk unsupported.

Fine motor and vision

Development of fine motor skills is dependent on gross motor and postural development as well as good vision. During the first 6 months of life a child will visually fix and track an object but lacks the manipulative skills to grasp it. These manipulative skills develop so that by 18 months the child can accurately reach out and pick up a small object with a pincer grip.

Speech and hearing

Hearing is paramount in the development of normal speech and language skills. The most common cause of delayed speech is hearing problems – all children with delayed speech development must have a hearing test arranged soon. Infants recognise and respond to voice – by 8 weeks a baby should 'still' to their mother's voice. Over the first year an infant will learn noises and intonation and may not produce any words but may babble with mature intonation. 'Dada' is usually the first 'word' as the 'da' sound is easier to produce than a 'ma'. From 1 year the number of words increases with the child putting words together by 2 years.

Social

Human social behaviour and interaction is extremely complicated and needs to be learnt by a developing child. Initially a baby will produce a social smile by 8 weeks to all humans. Over the first year an infant will develop social interaction with all humans but towards the end of the first year will start to develop 'stranger awareness' and will be anxious when not in the presence of a carer they recognise. After the first year the child starts to develop personal social skills such as feeding, dressing and continence. The development of social and interaction skills continues throughout childhood and schooling.

Table 3 Summary of the primitive reflexes

Reflex	Age at onset	Disappearance
Rooting	Birth	9 months
Palmar Grasp	Birth	Palm – 2–3 months Foot – 7-8 months
Galant	Few days after birth	7–8 days
Asymmetric Tonic Neck	1 month	3–5 months
Moro	Birth	2-3 months
Hand opening	Birth	2–3 months
Stepping	4 days	2 months
Placing	4 days	5–9 months

1.55 E

- Casting of objects: by 5 months
- Thumb and forefinger grasp: by 10 months
- Banging two cubes together: by 11 months
- Feed self with spoon: by 19 months
- Build tower of two cubes: by 20 months

See neurodevelopmental milestones (page 147).

1.56 D

The National Institute for Health and Clinical Excellence (NICE) have produced national guidelines for the management of head injuries. They are a little more complicated in children for a number of reasons. Children tend to vomit after injury; this may not be a result of a significant brain injury but a response to the injury. CT (investigation of choice for significant head injuries) requires a degree of cooperation and lying still, which may be difficult for younger children (< 5 years). In this patient, where there was loss of consciousness and some post-event vomiting, a CT scan may be indicated. However, as the child is 3 years old this may be difficult, unless it is performed under general anaesthetic. In these patients admission for neurological observation is preferable; if there is any decrease in GCS or development of focal neurological signs then CT is definitely indicated.

1.57 D

See neurodevelopmental milestones in answer to Question 1.54 (page 147).

1.58 D

Pure-tone audiometry is performed by placing headphones on the child and playing tones of various frequencies and intensities through them. The test requires a degree of cooperation, which should be present in a 5-year-old. Otoacoustic emissions (measuring the sound 'echo' from the cochlear) are a useful screening test, but they cannot distinguish between conductive and sensory deficits. Brainstem-evoked responses (measuring brain-wave response to auditory stimulus) can be performed at any age but is a lengthy test. The distraction test is routinely performed by health visitors at 8 months of age.

1.59 E

This is indeed the natural course of a capillary haemangioma. It is important that parents are told that there is a chance that the birthmark may never completely resolve.

1.60 D

All these investigations are useful when making the diagnosis. Once the diagnosis has been made, the investigation that has the biggest impact on management is for ANAs. There is a close correlation between being ANA positive and development of iridocyclitis (which can lead to blindness). ANA-positive children must have close ophthalmological follow-up.

1.61 A

The basal–bolus system involves a dose of long-acting insulin with three doses of short-acting insulin per day to coincide with meals, allowing greater flexibility with eating times and amounts (this is easier with older children). The long-acting insulin ensures a background level that provides more stable glycaemic control. This is ideally the best regimen for any child with diabetes. However, a 3-year-old child is unlikely to conform to the 'set' three meals per day and will tend to 'graze' (ie take small frequent bits of food). Given this eating behaviour, a regimen where there is a more constant level of insulin in the bloodstream is appropriate. Therefore, a twice-daily regimen is more likely to provide better control; indeed in some children whose eating patterns are so erratic a once-a-day injection of a long-acting insulin provides the best control.

1.62 D

Iron deficiency is the most likely because there is a microcytic anaemia with a low serum ferritin. The most likely cause of this in the UK is dietary deficiency. Chronic helminth infection is a common cause worldwide. Folate deficiency leads to megaloblastic anaemia. As the Hb electrophoresis shows 98% HbA (normal) then α-thalassaemia is ruled out.

1.63 E

As there is no 'mucosal' bleeding (ie lips/gums/tongue, urine or bowel) there is a lower risk of serious intracranial bleeding. There is no need to treat the lower risk groups acutely. The parents should have the diagnosis explained to them and the child should have frequent reviews. The natural course is that the average time to normal platelet numbers is 1 month; most others will be normal by 6 months but a small proportion will have chronic ITP. If there is mucosal bleeding there may be an increased risk of intracranial bleeding and active treatment may be advised.

1.64 C

The first tooth (normally lower incisor) erupts from 6 months onwards. There may be some symptoms of teething before this but this would be unusual at 4-and-a-half months. Many illnesses are attributed to teething; however, around this time there is a decline in maternal circulating antibodies. If there is any evidence that the infant is underfed (which should be picked up on examination) increased milk intake is advised because current advice is that weaning shouldn't start until 6 months. At around 4 months there is a recognised 'stormy period' associated with the development of new skills and physical growth.

1.65 D

This 5-year-old had a persistent cough that was characteristically nocturnal, accompanied by vomiting and with no evidence of any diurnal respiratory symptoms. The cough is related to the supine posture, especially as there was accompanying vomiting, which was a constant feature. Therefore in the first instance, the least invasive and most useful investigation is an ambulatory oesophageal pH study. A barium meal involves radiation, is not physiological and is indicated only if the possibility of a hiatus hernia is considered. A bronchoscopy and CT may be indicated if the initial investigations are negative.

1.66 D

There is no immediate risk to the child that would necessitate the police being called. Hospital security has no power to stop someone discharging him- or herself. The general practitioner might well be able to check on the baby but there is a need to inform Social Services. There are child protection risk factors for this baby – the maternal substance use and the father's behaviour – so Social Services clearly need to be informed.

1.67 A

This clinical picture fits with cardiac failure. Myocarditis is an important cause of acquired heart failure. The infective causes are commonly Coxsackie virus, influenza and adenoviruses, and bacterial causes as seen with *Borrelia burgdorferi* (Lyme disease). Rheumatic fever is unlikely if the ASOT is normal. A pancarditis may occur as part of Kawasaki's disease; however, this is unlikely to present in failure.

1.68 C

The twins are dehydrated, having lost a significant proportion of their birthweight. Exclusively breast-feeding the twins is obviously the ideal; however, this requires a lot of support, without which it may be unrealistic. Mothers should be encouraged to feed their babies by breast and supplement with formula if necessary. It is important that mothers should not be made to feel guilty for supplementing. In the situation above, there is most probably an insufficient intake. The best way of rehydrating most children is enterally – intravenous fluids would not be necessary in this situation. Bottle-feeding, either expressed breast milk or formula, would be reasonable; however, this might make it difficult for the mother to continue breast-feeding, an aim that should be supported. Nasogastric formula is a good initial method of reydration that allows breast-feeding to be supported.

PAPER 2 ANSWERS

Multiple Choice Answers

2.1 A

Below 16 years of age, consent of a parent or guardian is required, unless emergency treatment is required (when consent from a person *in loco parentis* is also unnecessary), or the child has given consent and the doctor considers that the child is of sufficient understanding to make an informed decision about medical care (including oral contraception) and the child refuses to allow the parents to be asked.

If a child aged under 16 years refuses surgery it can still be carried out if the doctor believes that the child doesn't have sufficient understanding to make an informed decision or if a court has considered the child's objection and told the doctor to proceed.

A mother and father have equal parental responsibilities for their legitimate child. If parents disagree it is probably inappropriate to proceed, although only one parent is needed for consent. An unmarried father is only financially responsible for his child; he has no intrinsic rights. (See answer 1.47.)

2.2 A, C, D

Acne affects 90% of teenagers and 25% of infants. Boys are more commonly affected than girls and acne persists beyond the age of 25 in 15%. Acne is usually associated with normal levels of testosterone. Causes include medications (eg oral contraceptive pill, steroids, phenytoin), irritants (eg cosmetics), occlusion (eg friction by head bands), emotional stress, menstruation and endocrine abnormalities (eg Cushing syndrome, diabetes, virilising tumour, polycystic ovaries).

Propionibacterium acnes is an anaerobic diphtheroid and this, together with yeast, colonises the blocked sebaceous glands and breaks down the sebum, releasing free fatty acids that cause an inflammatory reaction in the dermis. Secondary infection of the papules causes pustules, cysts and scars.

answers

In moderate cases, the treatment with erythromycin should continue for at least 6–12 months because its maximum effect is not achieved before 3–6 months. Even so, it may still relapse, requiring a further 3 months of treatment, so the patient must be well motivated. Severe cases (multiple cysts, pits, scars and keloids) and resistant moderate cases should be referred to the dermatologist. Roaccutane should be prescribed only by the hospital specialist. LFTs and lipids should be checked before starting treatment and monitored throughout. Roaccutane causes dry skin and mucosa and is 100% teratogenic (so oral contraception should be continued for at least 1 month after cessation of treatment).

2.3   A, B, E

A facial petechial rash may be a sign of smothering, although it may also be present in whooping cough. A generalised petechial rash should, however, raise suspicion of idiopathic thrombocytopenic purpura or meningococcal septicaemia. Multiple bruising on the shins of a 7-year-old boy is a normal finding, but bruising over the face, upper arms, wrists or inner thighs (with or without grip marks) in a child aged less than 9 months is of concern. A mongolian blue spot is commonly mistaken for abuse, but is in fact a harmless congenital blue marking, frequently occurring over the buttocks and sacrum.

Other superficial features compatible with physical child abuse include bite marks, a torn frenulum (from, for example, forced bottle-feeding), lacerations, ligature marks, burns and scalds. Bony injuries include metaphyseal or epiphyseal fractures, which raise suspicion of a twisting or pulling injury. Also, multiple fractures at different stages of healing or delayed presentation of fractures needs very careful assessment.

2.4   A, C, D

Turner's syndrome affects 1 in 2500 women. It has the genotype XO and mosaicism may occur with the genotype XO or XX. Note that testicular feminisation has the genotype XY. Features apparent at birth include a webbed neck, low posterior hairline and widely spaced nipples. Other features include a 'shield-shaped' chest, coarctation of the aorta, left heart defects, cubitus valgus, short stature (< 130 cm), hyperconvex nails, nystagmus, 'streak' ovaries – rudimentary or absent – and an association with Crohn's disease.

Somatotrophin is a useful treatment for short stature but only before the epiphyses have fused. Counselling is also an important part of the treatment and should cover genetic, medical and infertility issues.

2.5   B, D

Molluscum contagiosum is a pox DNA virus infection that typically presents as small, pearly, umbilicated lesions anywhere on the body, with characteristic satellite spread around the original lesion. The incubation period is 2–7 weeks and it spreads easily to siblings (eg via bath water) and the child remains infectious as long as the lesions are present. Atopic and immunocompromised children are particularly susceptible. The treatment of choice is patience because spontaneous resolution is the rule, typically after several months. Removal with phenol or liquid nitrogen is generally reserved for cosmetic reasons only.

2.6   B, E

Both irritant and contact dermatitis spare the flexures and should be treated by exposure to fresh air as much as is possible, frequent nappy changes, careful cleansing with baby lotion and routine use of barrier creams (eg zinc/castor oil). Secondary infection may be treated initially with a local antiseptic or antimicrobial. Candidiasis presents as a red rash with satellite lesions and shallow ulcers, and lesions on the skin should be treated with antifungal cream and white oral/mucosal lesions with gel.

Nappy rashes do not commonly become secondarily infected with *Staphylococcus aureus*. However, if there is impetiginous crusting or bullae, it must be considered. Topical antibiotics may be sufficient treatment if the infection is localised to the nappy area. If nappy rash fails to settle with the use of emollients while bathing and aqueous creams afterwards, then 0.5–1% hydrocortisone may be applied to the face and intertriginous areas. Potent fluorinated steroids (ie Dermovate) should be used only on thicker areas for less than 2–4 weeks and only if treatment with mild-to-moderate steroids has been unsuccessful.

Seborrhoeic dermatitis is an erythematous greasy rash, which commonly involves the nappy area, the occipital region and behind the ears. It may become secondarily infected with *Candida* spp., requiring treatment with antifungals.

2.7   A, D, E

Factitious or induced illness, previously termed 'Munchausen syndrome by proxy', refers to signs or symptoms in a child deliberately fabricated or induced by an adult. The child may be normal or have an illness and is usually of pre-school age. Although no organic cause can be found for the symptoms and all investigations are normal, the child may well show evidence of emotional abuse and/or failure to thrive. It is associated with a mortality rate of 2–10%.

The perpetrator is usually the mother and rarely the father, often with some kind of medical knowledge or training (eg nurse). The mother may not have a formal psychiatric diagnosis, but often has a personality disorder with maladaptation in other areas. She may have been abused herself as a child and subsequently seeks the attention of carers or refuge from other problems. Confrontation with evidence, while involving the partner, is a key part of the management, and this should be done in a sympathetic manner. Management should be discussed with Social Services and a strategy or case conference should be organised to consider the child's welfare, who should stay with the family if at all possible. Further help should be offered in the form of counselling, psychiatric referral and family/behavioural therapy.

2.8   A, C

There is a male:female ratio of 2:1. The feet are held in equinovarus (ie downwards and inwards) and club foot is associated with spina bifida. Initial management begins within 1 week of birth with splinting, where the deformity is 'over-corrected'. The infant then has weekly foot manipulations and, if the foot has not corrected by about 3 months, operative reduction or tendon release and fixation may be necessary.

answers

2.9   B, C, E

Cleft palate is equally prevalent (and is increasing in incidence) in boys and girls. Cleft lip is more common in boys, affects 1 in 750 live births and is associated with cleft palate in approximately 50% of cases. The risk to a child with one affected sibling is 5% and to one with two affected siblings 9%.

2.10   E

Tonsillectomy is indicated in children who have more than four attacks of acute tonsillitis a year, causing significant systemic illness, interference with growth, and school absences, recurrent cervical adenitis or peritonsillar abscess. It is associated with significant morbidity and mortality and should be performed only if clinically indicated and not at the request of the parents.

Although swallowing is uncomfortable, this does not lead to complete dysphagia postoperatively. Other complications include primary haemorrhage, occurring within 24 h, and usually caused by an inadequately ligated/cauterised vessel, and secondary haemorrhage, which is commonly the result of infection and occurs in 1% of patients about 1 week after the procedure. Quinsy (peritonsillar abscess) is a complication of tonsillitis and not tonsillectomy.

2.11   A, C, E

Wilms' nephroblastoma is the most common of all childhood malignant tumours accounting for 10% of cases. It presents before 5 years of age in 80% of children (median age 3.5 years), 95% are unilateral and 20% have metastasised at presentation, mainly to the lung and liver; 80% present with an abdominal mass, 25% with haematuria and about 30% with flank pain. Other features include failure to thrive and hemihypertrophy. Wilms' nephroblastoma may be sporadic, but, when familial, may be associated with aniridia, genitourinary malformations and retardation (WAGR syndrome). The gene for Wilms' tumour is found on chromosome 11.

Investigations of choice include intravenous urethrogram (renal pelvis distortion, hydronephrosis), ultrasonography and computed tomography (CT). Renal biopsy should be avoided. Treatment involves nephrectomy, chemotherapy (eg actinomycin E) and radiotherapy, which can be curative (80% 5-year survival rate).

2.12 C, E

Undescended testis occurs in 2–3% of term male neonates but in 15–30% of pre-term babies. Only 25% of cases are bilateral. A truly undescended testis will lie anywhere along the path of descent from the abdominal cavity. Other sites include the perineum, femoral region or base of the penis. Orchidopexy must be performed before 2 years of age to preserve function, preferably at 1 year. There is an increased incidence of torsion and also neoplasia (eg seminoma), which persists despite surgery.

2.13 A, D, E

Common side effects of sodium valproate include gastric irritation, nausea, ataxia and tremor, hyperammonaemia, increased appetite and weight gain, and transient hair loss (regrowth may be curly), plus impaired liver function and rarely pancreatitis. Stevens–Johnson syndrome is a typical side effect of phenytoin and hyperactivity is usually associated with clonazepam and phenobarbital, sodium valproate being more commonly linked with drowsiness.

2.14 A, B, C, D, E

Infection with the parainfluenza viruses and rhinovirus is particularly likely to precipitate an acute asthma attack.

2.15 C, E

High-risk infants do not require skin testing before immunisation up to the age of 3 months. BCG should be given only after a negative tuberculin test. It can be given at the same time as other live vaccines; otherwise a gap of 3 weeks should be observed. There is a risk that a suboptimal response to both may occur if this gap is not observed. Live oral polio vaccine (OPV), which works by inducing gut immunity, is the exception and can be given at any time. HIV infection is an absolute contraindication to BCG immunisation.

answers

2.16 B, E

The fetus is most at risk in the first 16 weeks of gestation, with approximately 55% affected if maternal infection occurs in the first 4 weeks. Cataract is associated with infection at 8–9 weeks, deafness at 5–7 weeks (although it may occur with second trimester infection) and cardiac lesions at 5–10 weeks. Other features include purpura, jaundice, hepatosplenomegaly, microcephaly, microphthalmia, retinopathy, developmental delay, cerebral palsy and thrombocytopenia. Miscarriage or stillbirth may also occur.

2.17 B, C

The 'incidence' is the number of new cases occurring during a specified period in a defined population, whereas the 'prevalence' is the number of cases at any particular time or during a specified period of time in a defined population. Therefore, an acute illness will have a high incidence, but a low prevalence, whereas the annual incidence of a chronic illness will be much lower than its prevalence. Both are expressed as a rate per 1000 of the population. The NMR is the number of deaths of live-born babies aged up to 1 month per 1000 live births and the IMR is the number of deaths of all infants aged under 1 year per 1000 live births.

2.18 A, D, E

Apgar scores (Table 4) are usually recorded at 1 min, 5 min and 5-min intervals after birth.

Table 3 The parameters for Apgar scores

Score	Pulse	Respiratory rate	Muscle tone	Reflex on suction	Colour
0	0	Nil	Limp	Nil	White
1	< 100	Slow/irregular	Limp/flexion	Grimace	Blue
2	> 100	Regular	Active	Cough	Pink

2.19 A, B, D, E

Depression may often initially present with various psychosomatic symptoms (eg abdominal pain, headache). However, the presence of an actual chronic physical disease (eg asthma, diabetes) is a predisposing factor and various medications, including steroids and some anticonvulsants, can result in depression. Depression may also present with behavioural problems such as vandalism or drug abuse, and younger children may regress, resulting in, for example, secondary enuresis.

2.20 B, D, E

At birth, 1% of hips are found to be unstable, more commonly on the left (60%) with one in five being bilateral. Risk factors include female sex (80%), family history, breech delivery, first child and history of oligohydramnios. Screening involves the Ortolani–Barlow manoeuvre with ultrasonography of suspicious joints, which shows the shape of the cartilaginous socket and position of the femoral head (radiographs are unhelpful before 6 weeks). If these tests are positive, neonates should be splinted in abduction for 6–12 weeks with clinical and radiological follow-up at 3, 6 and 12 months. Most hips will have stabilised with conservative methods; however, persistent instability will need surgery. This is more likely if initial treatment was delayed.

2.21 A, B, C, D, E

A prolonged neonatal jaundice caused by conjugated hyperbilirubinaemia is a known presenting feature of cystic fibrosis and should be investigated. However, a sweat test may be difficult to do in neonates, so alternative tests may be necessary (eg immune reactive trypsin). Any child with failure to thrive or short stature, especially if associated with respiratory or gastrointestinal symptoms, should also be investigated for cystic fibrosis. Pancreatic enzyme and dietary supplements are needed and may have to be increased when the child is ill (overnight tube feeding may be of benefit). Chest infections are common and cause progressive lung damage (ie bronchiectasis). The usual pathogens isolated are *Haemophilus influenzae*, *S. aureus*, and *Klebsiella* and *Pseudomonas* spp. Treatment includes chest physiotherapy, intravenous antibiotics and nebulised bronchodilators.

answers

2.22 B, C

Roseola infantum is a common disease of infancy. It commonly results from human herpesvirus (HHV) type 6 (HHV7 is also a likely pathogen). It has an incubation period of about 5–15 days, and then typically presents with a high fever for 3–4 days that subsides as a fine maculopapular rash, which develops initially on the torso before becoming widespread. It resolves in 2–3 days.

Human parvovirus type B19 is the cause of 'fifth disease', which is also known as the 'slapped-cheek' syndrome and erythema infectiosum. Roseola infantum is also known as 'sixth disease' and its only significant complication is febrile convulsions. Measles and chickenpox are associated with pneumonia.

2.23 A, B, C

Homocystinuria is a metabolic disorder associated with tall stature. Endocrine disorders resulting in tall stature include hyperthyroidism, precocious puberty and growth hormone excess (pituitary gigantism). Endocrine disorders resulting in short stature include pseudohypoparathyroidism, growth hormone deficiency, hypopituitarism, hypothyroidism and Cushing syndrome.

2.24 C, D, E

Cromoglicate is ineffective in the treatment of acute asthma but, although it has some effect as a preventive drug, as a result of various factors it has been omitted from the most recent British Thoracic Society (BTS) asthma guidelines. Inhalers deliver less than 5% of the drug to the lungs and even nebulisers only deliver less than 10%. Aminophylline can be used in the management of an acute attack; however, the loading dose should be omitted if the child is already on oral theophylline and ideally the drug level should be measured before the infusion is commenced. Regular low-dose inhaled steroids do not result in growth retardation. The incidence of oral candidiasis can be reduced if steroids are inhaled via a spacer device and rinsing the mouth afterwards reduces the risk further.

2.25 B, C, E

Primary prevention is aimed at preventing the 'accident' from happening and includes speed limits, stair gates, teaching road safety and child-proof catches on cupboards, whereas secondary prevention aims to prevent injury should the 'accident' happen and includes cycling helmets, seat belts, smoke alarms and fire extinguishers kept in the house. Child-resistant lids are a form of primary prevention because they prevent the child from reaching the drug, although blister packs for prescription drugs merely limit the number of tablets that a child can get at in a given time and are therefore a form of secondary prevention. Tertiary prevention aims to limit the impact of an injury once the 'accident' has happened and includes teaching parents first aid skills and providing good access to the emergency services.

2.26 A, B, E

The Dubowitz system is a system for estimating the gestational age of neonates from 26 to 44 weeks. It includes various neurological criteria (eg posture, head lag) and physical (or external) criteria, which include: presence of oedema; skin texture; skin colour (not crying); skin opacity (trunk); lanugo (over back); plantar creases; nipple formation; breast size; ear form and firmness; and development of genitalia (ie presence of testes in scrotum).

2.27 A, B, C

Infants born to mothers with poorly controlled diabetes may have sacral agenesis, hypomagnesaemia, hypocalcaemia, polycythaemia and Erb's palsy secondary to the increased risk of shoulder dystocia.

2.28 C, E

Trimethoprim is usually the best first-line antibiotic, because *E. coli* (responsible for 80% of UTIs) is often resistant to amoxicillin. Augmentin, nitrofurantoin and cephalosporins are also useful. Trimethoprim and nitrofurantoin are often used for prophylaxis in children with vesicoureteric reflux (VUR), and are effective when given once daily. Prevention of UTIs includes the avoidance of constipation, ensuring the bladder is completely empty after voiding and wiping in a front-to-back direction in girls. If there is no evidence of chronic pyelonephritis then treatment of asymptomatic bacteriuria is not recommended because it may allow a virulent strain to reinfect with the elimination of an avirulent one. Surgery may be necessary if the UTI is secondary to calculi, obstruction or severe VUR with failed medical management.

2.29 B, E

Cerebral palsy is a disorder of posture and movement resulting from a non-progressive lesion of the developing brain before or during the neonatal period. The expression of the lesion changes as the brain matures. It has a prevalence of 2.5 in 1000. Learning disability occurs in < 50% of children. Other associated disabilities include visual (25%), language (90%) and hearing loss (25%). The importance of the various causes of cerebral palsy is controversial. Perinatal insult is now thought to be less important as an aetiological factor. Other causes include cryptogenic (35%), genetic (20%), postnatal disease, eg meningitis (20%), and intrauterine infection, irradiation or drug-induced damage (5%). Diagnosis of cerebral palsy in babies aged under 6 months may be difficult unless it is severe. Similarly, mild cases may present only with delayed developmental milestones or clumsiness.

2.30 A

The stepwise treatment of asthma involves starting at the 'step' most appropriate for the severity and moving up or down as needed. Treatment can be gradually 'stepped down' if control has been good for over 6 months.

- Step 1: as requires inhaled bronchodilators
- Step 2: + low-dose inhaled corticosteroids
- Step 3: + long-acting inhaled β agonists
- Step 4: + high-dose inhaled corticosteroids, oral leukotriene antagonists and/or theophylline
- Step 5: + oral corticosteroids.

2.31 A

Asthma affects > 10% of children and causes approximately 50 deaths per year in the UK. Most are teenagers with chronic severe asthma. The prevalence has been gradually increasing over the past 20 years. This may be as a result of increased parental awareness, pollution and changing infant feeding patterns. The mortality rate has, however, remained static.

2.32 A, B, E

The gene for cystic fibrosis is located on the long arm of chromosome 7 and analysis of fetal DNA obtained in the first trimester (at chorionic villous sampling) will confirm the diagnosis. The gene carrier rate is 1 in 22 of the white population and about 75–80% of these gene mutations in the UK are caused by a deletion at ΔF508, although this frequency varies geographically (eg in Italy, it is responsible for only about 40% of mutations). Cystic fibrosis is an autosomal recessive disorder, so two carrier parents have a 1 in 2 chance of having a carrier child, a 1 in 4 chance of having a normal child and a 1 in 4 chance of having an affected child.

2.33 A, C

Generalised 'absences' present between 3 and 13 years and are more common in girls. 'Absences' characteristically last less than 10 s and recur more than 10 times a day. There is no collapse and the patient is usually unaware of them. Affected children have a normal IQ but may have learning difficulties secondary to the frequency of the attacks. The EEG shows a bilateral, symmetrical, 3 Hz spike-and-wave pattern, which may be precipitated by hyperventilation (EEG spike waves over rolandic ones are typical of simple partial seizures). CT reveals no structural abnormality and the cause is unknown, although they may have a familial predisposition. It usually remits in adult life, but 30% go on to develop generalised tonic–clonic epilepsy. First-line treatment is with valproate or ethosuximide.

2.34 A, C, D

Constipation is the passage of hard, dry stools resulting in distress for the child. However, it may present as diarrhoea when constipation with overflow is present. Breast-fed babies may pass infrequent soft stools (eg weekly), but this is a normal variation and parents should be reassured. Constipation is most commonly secondary to a low-fibre diet and other causes, including medication, dehydration anal trauma (eg postoperative, abuse) and spinal disorders (eg spina bifida). Mental disability is associated with failure to develop a regular bowel habit; however, Down's syndrome is also associated with an increased incidence of Hirschsprung's disease.

2.35 C, D, E

The Butler-Schloss report recommends that parents should be invited to attend all or part of the conference, unless the chairperson feels that their presence will be detrimental to the child's interests. Ideally a case conference should be held with parental consent/involvement without an EPO being necessary. However, if an EPO is necessary, this may be a convenient time to have the conference. A senior officer from social services must act as the chairperson. Other invitees include the GP, paediatrician, police child protection team, a solicitor from the local authority and other specialists as appropriate. The case conference acts in an advisory capacity only and considers the evidence of abuse, the cause, the risk of recurrence and safety of any siblings. However, apart from deciding whether to put the child on the Child Protection Register, all other decisions are made by the directors of Social Services, who will obviously take into consideration the findings of the case conference.

Answers to Extended Matching Questions

2.36 Choice of investigations

1   H – Haemoglobin electrophoresis

The most likely cause of dactylitis in a 6-month-old child is sickle cell disease. The investigation that would diagnose this is Hb electrophoresis.

2   B – Bone marrow aspiration cytology

The most likely cause for this is immune thrombocytopenic purpura (ITP); however, aplastic anaemia is possible, as is ALL. Bone marrow aspiration cytology is the investigation that would give a definitive diagnosis.

3   I – Monospot

A 14-year-old boy with this history is most likely to have glandular fever; a monospot would diagnose this definitively.

answers

2.37 Decisions about life-saving treatment

1   B – The 'no chance' situation

2   E – The 'unbearable' situation

3   C – The 'no purpose' situation

The RCPCH issued guidelines in 1997 on when it could be considered appropriate to 'withdraw or withhold lifesaving treatment'. The five situations are as follows:

1.   Brain-dead child: the formal criteria for brain death are met.

2.   PVS: the formal criteria for PVS are met.

3.   'No chance' situation: despite all treatments, there is no chance of the child surviving, so it could be considered that withdrawal of care is appropriate.

4.   'No purpose' situation: a child may survive given the necessary interventions but will be so impaired that he or she will probably not achieve 'personhood' or be able to make decisions about his or her own life.

5.   'Unbearable' situation: the treatment is so invasive and has so many side effects that it may be more than the child can bear (the treatment is worse than the disease).

It is important to note that withdrawing and withholding treatment from children should be done as part of a multidisciplinary process with full parental involvement.

2.38 Heart defects

1   E – Innocent (flow) murmur

This is an incidental finding in a presumably acyanotic, otherwise healthy 3-year-old. The murmur is soft, ejection systolic at the LSE only, and so a flow murmur is the most likely diagnosis (a result of the increased flow because the child is unwell). The GP should re-examine once this acute illness has resolved.

2   F – PDA

This is not a cyanotic lesion. As she is only 12 hours old the most likely diagnosis is a PDA that has yet to close. Full femoral pulses are usually felt in a PDA.

3   B – ASD

Again this is an acyanotic lesion. The murmur heard is a pulmonary flow murmur resulting from the increased flow. The flow through the defect itself is not great enough (as atrial) to produce a murmur. A fixed split of the second heart sound is classic of an ASD. Hepatomegaly is a characteristic sign of heart failure in infants and small children.

2.39 Common infections

1 D – Epstein–Barr virus (EBV)

Glandular fever should always be considered in older children with sore throats. If amoxicillin is given when a child has EBV infection, it will cause a florid maculopapular rash. This is one way of making the diagnosis!

2 C – Coxsackie virus A16

Vesicles on the hands and feet, and probably in the mouth if refusing food, are the reason why hand, foot and mouth disease has that name. It is caused by Coxsackie virus A16 and is very contagious. Nurseries often close during an outbreak.

3 F – *Mycoplasma pneumoniae*

Target lesions are seen in erythema multiforme. In an unwell child with erythema multiforme mycoplasma infection should always be considered, as must herpes simplex infection. Stevens–Johnson syndrome is an important complication.

answers

2.40 Statistics and research methods

1   **C – Lead time**

2   **E – Likelihood ratio**

3   **J – Specificity**

- Lead time: the time between a condition being identified by screening and a condition becoming clinically apparent.

- Lag time: the time between an intervention being assessed as clinically useful and an intervention actually entering everyday practice.

- Sensitivity: percentage of those with a condition who correctly test positive.

- Specificity: percentage of those without a condition who correctly test negative.

- Likelihood ratio: odds of a positive test result in an affected individual compared with a positive result in an unaffected individual – this is a positive likelihood ratio.

- Number needed to treat (NNT): the number of patients who would need to have an intervention for a set outcome to be shown in one of them.

- Prevalence: the total number of cases in a population at any one time (expressed as a proportion of the total population).

- Incidence: rate at which new cases of a condition occur in a population (over a set period of time – usually 1 year).

answers

2.41 Immediate interventions

1   J – Vagal manoeuvres

Any child in SVT should have vagal manoeuvres tried first because they are quick and easy (and can be effective). The strategies that can be used are: an older child can try a Valsalva manoeuvre by blowing up a balloon. Infants can have their face immersed in cold water to try to elicit a diving reflex. Unilateral carotid massage can also be tried.

2   I – Synchronous DC shock – 0.5 J/kg

The low saturations and prolonged capillary refill indicate that the child is in shock. A shocked child in VT but with a pulse should undergo asynchronous DC cardioversion at an initial power of 0.5 J/kg (performed after rapid sequence induction anaesthesia). The underlying diagnosis is likely to be a tricyclic antidepressant overdose.

3   E – Asynchronous DC shock – 4 J/kg

Treatment of VF/pulseless VT is with asynchronous DC shock of 4 J/kg (followed by a further 4 J/kg, then 4 J/kg). Cardiopulmonary resuscitation (CPR) must continue when the shocks are not being given, and it is important to give epinephrine (adrenaline) – but only DC shock will convert the rhythm to sinus. This is the 2005 Resuscitation Council UK guidelines (previously 2J /kg, 2 J/kg, 4 J/kg).

(All these answers are taken from *Advanced Paediatric Life Support – The practical approach*, 3rd edn. London: BMJ Books, 2001, and relevant updates from the ALSG (Advanced Life Support Group) and Resuscitation Council UK.)

2.42 Neoplasms

1   B – Acute lymphoblastic leukaemia

ALL is the most common malignancy in childhood (35–40% of all childhood malignancies). The incidence is highest in early childhood. Diagnosis is made on bone marrow aspiration; however, blast cells can often be seen in the peripheral blood. The treatment generally lasts for around 2 years. Survival rates are as high as 85% at 5 years.

2   J – Wilms' tumour

There are only two likely diagnoses in this case: Wilms' nephroblastoma or neuroblastoma. As there is blood in the urine then there is probably renal involvement and therefore a Wilms' nephroblastoma is the more likely of the two.

For further details see answer to Question 2.11 (page 159). Both Wilms' nephroblastomas and neuroblastomas count for 8% each of all childhood malignancies.

3   G – Non-Hodgkin's lymphoma

This is a typical history for non-Hodgkin's lymphoma. The shortness of breath is caused by mediastinal involvement (which can ultimately cause superior vena cava [SVC] obstruction). The staging and treatment of non-Hodgkin's lymphoma are essentially the same as in adults. Lymphomas count for 15% of all childhood malignancies and are the second most common solid tumours after the central nervous system (CNS) tumours. The other childhood malignancies are bone tumours (7%), retinoblastoma (2%), and others such as rhabdomyosarcoma or adenocarcinoma.

2.43 Antimicrobial therapy

1   C – Intravenous cefotaxime 100 mg/kg

This is presumed meningococcal sepsis until proven otherwise.

A high-dose, intravenous, broad-spectrum antibiotic must be given as soon as possible – intravenous ceftriaxone is a commonly used antibiotic, but should be given at high dose of 80 mg/kg.

2   G – Intravenous cefotaxime 50 mg/kg

The most likely diagnosis is group B streptococcal (GBS) sepsis, which is highly sensitive to penicillin – the treatment of choice. However, it would not be used as a monotherapy because there is minimal Gram-negative cover. Whether or not there is Gram-negative sepsis, GBS must be covered. The most appropriate broad-spectrum antibiotic in this list is intravenous cefotaxime, although the neonatal high dose is 50 mg/kg.

3   H – Oral ciprofloxacin

Children with cystic fibrosis who have a chest exacerbation but remain well will normally be treated with oral ciprofloxacin because it has good broad cover and excellent pseudomonal cover. If there are signs of respiratory distress or the child is unwell, admission and use of intravenous antibiotics (eg tobramycin) should be seriously considered.

Best of Five Answers

2.44 C

This is the law as it stands at present. The hand must be open (not a clenched fist), no implement may be used and 'no injury' inflicted (so it must leave no mark). It could well be argued that, even if no mark is left, an 'injury' may still have been inflicted.

2.45 B

Dietary advice is always an integral part of the management of constipation. A diet with adequate fibre, fruit and vegetables, and fluid intake should be encouraged. However, in this case some lactulose will help soften the stools to allow a normal bowel habit to be re-established. Senna would also achieve this but can cause stomach cramps and less compliance.

2.46 C

While all of the pieces of advice are valid, it is most important to advise that circumcision should not take place. Many parents are keen for circumcision for ethnic or religious reasons; however, circumcision can make a surgical hypospadias repair much more difficult.

2.47 B

Some of these investigations are more useful than others. Abdominal ultrasonography will detect the enlargement of abdominal/para-aortic lymph nodes but not help in establishing a diagnosis. A Paul Bunnell test, if positive, will establish a diagnosis, but this is unlikely given the history. CRP/LFTs and amylase may indicate an inflammatory process but again will not help establish a diagnosis. A blood film would be the most useful given the history (leukaemia, haematopoietic disorders).

177

2.48 E

Antibiotics are of limited benefit in the treatment of otitis media. They can shorten the duration of the illness but the number needed to treat is 17. Of the cases of otitis media, 80% resolve without treatment. Supportive measures such as antipyretics and analgesics are important measures to recommend to parents. (Glasziou PP, Del Mar CB, Sanders SL, Hayem M (2003) Antibiotics for acute otitis media in children (Cochrane Review). In: *Cochrane Library*, Issue 4.)

2.49 D

The initial cranial ultrasound scan in a 25/40 gestation infant is primarily to look for intraventricular haemorrhage, because the period in which it is most likely to happen is the initial 48 h. The other features are important but may well not be seen initially.

2.50 A

All of these are important elements of a prolonged jaundice screen. Biliary atresia is the important cause of conjugated hyperbilirubinaemia. It is surgically corrected by the Kasai procedure and this should be done before 60 days (8 weeks) of life, otherwise the outcome is markedly worse. TFTs are theoretically not so important to perform because the Guthrie test should screen for hypothyroidism. The other tests are not as urgent as the split bilirubin.

2.51 C

Enteral rehydration using an oral rehydration solution is almost invariably the preferred way of rehydrating children. If a child is not tolerating small frequent feeds nasogastric rehydration is an underused next best step. The fluid can be run through a continuous pump so that it is better tolerated. Intravenous fluids are effective but can have profound effects on the serum electrolyte balance if not monitored closely. Most children will tolerate fluids in an A&E department, but failure to take fluids orally is not an indication for intravenous therapy.

2.52 C

HBsAb +ve, HBeAg +ve is classified as high risk of infectivity to the infant. The babies in such cases should receive both the hepatitis B vaccine and hepatitis B immunoglobulin within the first 24 h of life. Low-risk infants (HBsAb +ve, HBeAg −ve) should receive hepatitis vaccine only.

2.53 C

- Brush teeth with help: by 26 months
- Play ball with examiner: by 17 months
- Wave bye-bye: by 15 months
- Put on a T-shirt unaided: by 3 years
- Play 'pat-a-cake': by 11 months.

See neurodevelopmental milestones in answer to Question 1.54 (page 147).

2.54 B

A star chart for dry nights is a useful tool for managing nocturnal enuresis. Simple measures such as minimising fluid intake before bed and ensuring that the child goes to the toilet before going to bed are important. Medical interventions are not a good first-line measure; desmopressin is effective but there is a high relapse rate off treatment. Imipramine is infrequently used now because there are more effective treatments and it has serious side effects. Enuresis clinics provide good support but most do not accept referrals for children aged under 7 years old.

2.55 C

- Able to run steadily: by 20 months
- Walk backwards: by 16 months
- Hop on one leg: by 4 years
- Walk up stairs unaided: by 20 months
- Throw ball overhand: by 3 years.

See neurodevelopmental milestones in answer to Question 1.54 (page 147).

answers

2.56 A

If the child is thought to be in immediate danger then a PPO is the quickest and most effective because it allows the child to be taken to a place of safety. An EPO court wardship and temporary fostering may occur later but not immediately. A section 47 meeting is convened by Social Services for the professionals and family to assess a child's needs and the ability of the current carer to ensure a safe and nurturing environment.

2.57 E

Femoral nerve block is a safe and very effective method of pain relief for limb injuries. The other options are, of course, useful but probably not sufficiently strong for this severity of injury. Splinting is vital but analgesia should be given first. Intravenous morphine should be used with caution if there is the possibility of a significant head injury. (*Advanced Paediatric Life Support*, 3rd edn – see answer to Question 2.41, page 174.)

2.58 A

Tuberous sclerosis – autosomal dominant, 1 in 50 000:

- 'Ash-leaf' macules (from infancy): depigmented lesions approximately 1–2 cm long
- 'Shagreen' patches (from 2 years): areas of roughened skin, usually sacral, likened to shark skin
- Adenoma sebaceum (from 5 years): 1- to 2-mm papules, usually facial (butterfly distribution)
- Epilepsy (usually before 2 years).

Neurofibromatosis type 1 – autosomal dominant, 1 in 2500:

- Café-au-lait spots (> 2 in children under 5 years, > 5 in children over 5 years significant)
- Axillary freckling
- Neurofibromas (from 12 years): papules anywhere on the body
- Epilepsy only in 10%.

Ataxia telangiectasia – autosomal recessive, a chromosomal repair defect. Affected children present as late walkers. Ataxia develops in early childhood and is progressive:

- Conjunctival telangiectasia: develops from 5 years

- Incontinentia pigmenti: X-linked dominant.

- Vesicular stage: neonatal period, linear distribution; resolves by 1 month

- Verrucose stage: 1–4 months, warty lesions appearing mainly on limbs; resolves by 6 months

- Whorl stage: by 2 years, linear and whorl pattern of hyperpigmentation on limbs

- Epilepsy in over 30%.

Sturge–Weber syndrome – sporadic, 1 in 50 000:

- Naevus in trigeminal distribution with an ipsilateral leptomeningeal haemangioma

- Intracranial calcification is common, especially in the occipital region

- Seizures develop in early childhood.

2.59 A

Minimal change disease is by far the most common cause of nephrotic syndrome in childhood. The next most common is focal segmental glomerular sclerosis. Finnish microcystic disease is a rare cause of nephrotic syndrome seen only in infancy.

2.60 D

The history and site of the pain are unlikely for appendicitis, mesenteric adenitis and pyelonephritis. A UTI is unlikely with no symptoms and a negative dipstick. A basal pneumonia is an important differential diagnosis in a febrile child who presents with abdominal pain.

2.61 B

This is a difficult situation and different practitioners may have different views. If there is a clear history of GOR then a trial of Gaviscon is simple and has minimal side effects, and is therefore a reasonable approach. If there is no improvement in the symptoms, further treatment can be initiated as warranted. There is an argument that, as the child is thriving, the GOR is something the child will outgrow, but is an indication for treatment in the interim. An oesophageal pH study is a good investigation for diagnosing severity of GOR, whereas a contrast upper GI study (or barium meal) is non-physiological and its main value here is in demonstrating a hiatus hernia; however, if there are good clinical features investigations may not be needed.

2.62 A

Five pills is not a toxic dose. As the overdose was within 1 h activated charcoal may reduce systemic absorption and is worth giving (if she will take it!). Levels for paracetamol and salicylate should be taken at 4 h to assess whether treatment is needed (because she may have concealed what and how much she actually took). All overdoses should, ideally, be discussed with the National Poisons Information Service (NPIS), especially if staggered overdose or more than one substance was taken. Most A&E departments now have online access to 'Toxbase', the NPIS website that allows quick referencing for overdose management.

2.63 C

Any child who has taken a deliberate overdose, even if no medical treatment is required, must be seen by a child psychiatrist. It is considered best practice not to discharge until assessed safe to do so by a child and adolescent psychiatrist. This means that most will be admitted until assessed, although some may be seen in A&E depending on the level of psychiatric service provided.

2.64 C

Isolated gross motor delay in a child with otherwise normal development must raise the question of muscular dystrophy. The most useful test in diagnosing this is a CK level. A detailed physiotherapy assessment would in all likelihood raise the question of muscular dystrophy but a CK would be needed to confirm it. Thyroid function testing is important in generalised developmental delay, but less so in this case. An MRI and EMG are unlikely to be helpful initially.

2.65 B

In the context of a normal blood pressure and only a trace of urine, there is little evidence of a severe nephritis needing renal biopsy. It would be unwise to discharge a child at this stage. The most appropriate monitoring is blood pressure and urine dipsticks until clear – this is non-invasive and can accurately monitor the development of nephritis.

2.66 D

Acute rheumatic fever is a very likely diagnosis with two to three minor features (fever, raised CRP and prolonged P–R interval) and two major features (flitting polyarthropathy and pericarditis) after an URTI. Acute myocarditis/pericarditis is one of the few indications for bed rest. High-dose aspirin is indicated; penicillin is often given, although of equivocal value in this situation. Diuretics are indicated only for cardiac failure and corticosteroids rather than ACTH are often given for prolonged fever and/or inflammation.

2.67 E

The most serious side effect of TCAs is the development of ventricular tachycardia. This child has a reduced conscious level, and is profoundly tachycardic, tachypnoeic and hypotensive; these would all be seen with VT and also the CNS effects of TCAs. β Blockers would more likely cause a bradycardia. Aspirin can cause an initial hyperventilation and then a metabolic acidosis.

answers

2.68 A

The history and examination are compatible with chronic fatigue syndrome (CFS), also known generally as myalgic encephalomyelitis (ME) or postviral fatigue syndrome. The only treatment for which there is some evidence base is graded mobilisation and physiotherapy. Increased rest is of no proven value and does not improve mobilisation and exercise tolerance. Home tuition may be advised, but the primary aim is gradual reintegration into school. Psychological input may be useful but is often resisted by parents who perceive this as primarily a medical/organic problem. Antidepressants are mainly indicated for an associated clinical depression.

PAPER 3 ANSWERS

Multiple Choice Answers

3.1 B, E

Glue ear causes a conductive hearing loss and the resulting deafness may present with behavioural problems as a result of the child's frustration. The natural history of the condition means that most children will have normal hearing by 8 years of age, regardless. However, early treatment is vital to ensure that the hearing is adequate for normal development. Surgical treatment involves myringotomy and insertion of grommets, which allow the middle ear to be ventilated – a role that is eventually resumed by the eustachian tube. Most grommets are extruded 2 months to 2 years after insertion.

3.2 A, E

Hib infection is rare before age 3 months; the incidence steadily rises, peaking at approximately 10–11 months and then declining to the age of 4 years. All children younger than 13 months should therefore receive the full immunisation course. From 13 months to 2 years non-immunised children should receive a single Hib dose with their MMR (children are less at risk in this age group and therefore a single dose is effective). The Hib vaccine is not live and is therefore safe in immunocompromised patients. Of invasive Hib disease, 60% presents as meningitis, 15% as epiglottitis, 10% as septicaemia alone and the remaining 15% includes septic arthritis, osteomyelitis, cellulitis, pneumonia and pericarditis. It has a mortality rate of about 2%.

3.3   A, D

Cardiac arrest in children has an extremely poor prognosis in most cases and is most frequently caused by severe illness or injury, resulting in hypoxia, acidosis and respiratory arrest. The few survivors often have neurological sequelae. However, cold water drowning is the one area where prolonged resuscitation after cardiac arrest has had some success. Finding the correct size of equipment during paediatric resuscitation can be confusing and the Breslow tape is extremely useful at removing the guesswork. From the height, it estimates the child's weight and each 'weight' has a list of appropriate drug dosages, fluid boluses and equipment sizes for easy reference. Cuffed endotracheal tubes are rarely used in children because, unlike adults, the narrowest diameter is at the level of the cricoid ring, which is susceptible to the pressure effects of the cuff. Intraosseous access is suitable in children aged up to 6 years and has been more recently accepted as a last resort in older children and adults (sternal intraosseous placement).

3.4   B

Between 0 and 1 year of age an infant should ideally have at least five recordings of weight and probably one or two recordings of length; between 1 and 2 years of age they should have at least three recordings and children aged over 2 years should be recorded annually. Measurements should be plotted on (new 9th) centile charts as part of a screen for growth failure. All children below the 2nd centile should be reviewed by the GP, especially if the child has tall parents. The GP should also review all children crossing a centile, even if still within normal limits or if there is parental concern. All children below the 0.4th centile should be referred for a specialist opinion. Normal growth velocity of children over 2 years is 5 cm/year and is calculated by the formula: [Increase in height in cm $\times$ 12]/[Number of months] = cm/year.

3.5 A, B, E

If a child has an unkempt, frightened, withdrawn appearance with 'frozen watchfulness' and, possibly, failure to thrive, developmental delay and evidence of physical injury, practitioners should have a high degree of suspicion of abuse. An acute hyphaema (ie blood in the anterior chamber of the eye) may result from serious shaking and scalds over both buttocks are typical of a forced immersion. However, a midclavicular fracture in a 10-day-old infant may have resulted from a difficult delivery and, although a green/yellow bruise is evidence of an old injury (more precise estimation from the colour of the bruise is notoriously unreliable), this is a common finding in an active toddler.

3.6 A, B

Tinea pedis (athlete's foot) is common in adolescents, leading to itchy, macerated and peeling skin between the toes with an unpleasant odour. Tinea capitis (scalp ringworm) is often caused by *Trichophyton* sp. and results in hair loss, circular patches of alopecia with scaling skin and broken hairs. Tinea corporis results in itching with or without scaly circular lesions anywhere on the skin. There may also be small vesicles at the periphery. The differential diagnosis includes eczema, psoriasis and the 'Herald patch' of pityriasis rosea. *Microsporum canis* infections fluoresce under Wood's light. Fungal infections are identified by examining skin scrapings and plucked hairs under the microscope for hyphae and spores.

Small areas may be treated with topical clotrimazole cream; however, large areas require a 4- to 6-week course of oral griseofulvin. The rest of the family (including pets) should be examined and treated as necessary.

3.7   B, C

One per cent of hips are found to be unstable at birth and are more common on the left (60%). Risk factors include female sex (80%), family history, breech delivery, first child and history of oligohydramnios. Screening involves the Ortolani–Barlow manoeuvre with ultrasonography of suspicious joints (radiographs are unhelpful before 6 weeks). If these tests are positive, neonates should be splinted in abduction for 6–12 weeks with clinical and radiological follow-up at 3, 6 and 12 months. Most hips will stabilise with conservative methods; however, those with persistent instability will need surgery, and is more likely if initial treatment was delayed.

3.8   A, B, C

Normal arterial pressure ($P\text{a}co_2$) is an ominous sign, because a patient with acute asthma usually hyperventilates and consequently has low $P\text{a}co_2$; however, it will also be normal in very mild asthma so it cannot be interpreted in isolation from the clinical assessment. A normal $P\text{a}co_2$ may imply that the patient is becoming exhausted and beginning to hypoventilate, and may indicate impending respiratory arrest as the $P\text{a}co_2$ continues to climb. The BTS (British Thoracic Society) guidelines define severe acute asthma as being: too breathless to talk, too breathless to feed, respirations > 50 breaths/min, pulse > 140 beats/min and a peak expiratory flow rate (PEFR) < 50% predicted or best. Other features of life-threatening asthma include PEFR < 33% predicted or best, a silent chest or poor respiratory effort, agitation, fatigue, decreased level of consciousness and central cyanosis. (Note that peripheral cyanosis is of little predictive value because it may be affected by numerous causes, including the weather!) Pulsus paradoxus of > 20 mmHg is said to indicate severe acute asthma, although this is a difficult sign to demonstrate and is rarely used. Pectus carinatum is, however, a sign of chronic asthma and has no significance with regard to the severity of an acute attack.

3.9 B, C

Acute epiglottitis is caused by *Haemophilus influenzae* type b. It generally occurs between 2 and 6 years of age, and the diagnosis is made from the history and classic clinical appearance. Within a few hours of developing a sore throat, the child becomes hot, toxic, drools as a result of difficulty swallowing, and is anxious and unable to speak . The child is dyspnoeic, has inspiratory stridor and subcostal recession, and typically holds the head in hyperextension to maximise the airway. There is usually no cough. Anything that may increase the child's distress should be avoided because this may precipitate a respiratory arrest requiring an emergency attempt at endotracheal intubation by junior staff. This would include unnecessary investigations, such as a lateral neck radiograph, and examination/instrumentation of the throat is absolutely contraindicated. If the condition is suspected an experienced anaesthetist should be called to perform an elective endotracheal intubation in a controlled environment, such as an operating theatre.

3.10 A, B, C, D, E

Common side effects of phenytoin include nausea, vomiting, mental confusion, dizziness, headache and tremor. Coarse facies, acne, hirsutism and gingival hyperplasia are particularly undesirable in adolescent patients. Rarer side effects include dyskinesias, SLE, erythema multiforme (Stevens–Johnson syndrome) and blood disorders. Plasma calcium may be lowered (rickets and osteomalacia). Ataxia, slurred speech, nystagmus and blurred vision are signs of overdosage.

3.11 B, C, E

Tics are defined as stereotypical, repetitive, involuntary movements. Simple developmental tics affect 15% of primary age schoolchildren (Years 1–6). They involve movements of the head, neck and shoulders (eg blinking, sniffing, shrugging) and are not generally of pathological significance. Most are usually outgrown by 4 years of age and rarely persist beyond adolescence. Tics may be familial in origin.

3.12 C, D

The most common reason for a child to be admitted to hospital in the UK is for an acute exacerbation of asthma. Initial investigations should include PEFR in children aged over 5 years; however, it is difficult to measure accurately in younger children and is therefore not a reliable measure of severity in this group. A chest radiograph is not required routinely and is indicated only if the diagnosis is in doubt or an associated severe infection or significant pneumothorax is clinically suspected. Intravenous steroids should be given with an acute exacerbation only if the child is vomiting; otherwise oral preparations are sufficient. Intravenous fluids should be restricted to two-thirds of normal maintenance, because increased secretion of antidiuretic hormone (ADH) occurs with severe asthma, resulting in fluid retention.

3.13 A, B, D, E

The MMR vaccine is contraindicated in patients who are allergic to neomycin or kanamycin. In children who have had a previous anaphylactic reaction to egg, immunisation is not absolutely contraindicated and should be discussed with a local paediatrician or immunisation coordinator. The MMR vaccine should not be given within 3 weeks of another live vaccine, because this results in a suboptimal response. Likewise, it is contraindicated in patients who have received an injection of immunoglobulin within 3 months, because no response will be mounted in the presence of immunoglobulin that may contain antibodies to measles, mumps or rubella. Pregnancy should be avoided for at least 1 month after immunisation, which may well result in a rash with or without fever from about day 5–10, lasting about 2 days. It is therefore sensible to provide advice on temperature control at the time of immunisation.

3.14 B, D, E

An adverse obstetric history is a risk factor including previous ectopic pregnancy, abortion, antepartum haemorrhage, pre-term labour, caesarean section, perinatal death and congenital abnormality. A birth interval of 18–36 months is associated with the lowest perinatal mortality rate, whereas an interval of less than 12 months has the highest rate. Multiple pregnancy and maternal age greater than 35 years are also risk factors.

3.15 A, C, E

Plagiocephaly is associated with craniosynostosis and also with babies who have suffered damage to their sternomastoid muscle and consequently develop a sternomastoid tumour (which may present with a torticollis that is present from birth). This pulls the head persistently to the affected side, resulting in retarded facial growth on that side and hence facial asymmetry. A recent increase in the incidence may be attributable to the 'back to sleep' campaign to combat sudden infant death syndrome (SIDS). Advice on alternating the head position in the cot generally results in spontaneous improvement over time. If it is secondary to sternomastoid tumour, it may also resolve, but it may need physiotherapy if it persists.

3.16 A, C, E

Common side effects of carbamazepine include nausea and vomiting, dizziness, drowsiness, headache, ataxia (phenytoin and clonazepam also have these effects), confusion and agitation (in elderly people), visual disturbances, anorexia, diarrhoea and constipation. A mild transient erythematous rash may occur in a large number of patients (this may need discontinuation of the drug if it worsens). Leukopenia and other blood disorders (thrombocytopenia, agranulocytosis and aplastic anaemia) are also recognised. Rickets is a known side effect of phenytoin and phenobarbital whereas transient hair loss is typical of sodium valproate.

3.17 A, C

Common side effects of clonazepam are somnolence (and paradoxical hyperactivity), muscle hypotonia, fatigue, dizziness, coordination disturbances and hypersalivation in infancy. Rarer side effects include blood disorders and abnormal liver function. Acne occurs with phenytoin and nystagmus with overdose. Reversible leukopenia is more typical of carbamazepine.

3.18 A, C, D, E

Cystic fibrosis is an autosomal recessive disorder and affects approximately 1 in 2000 live births in the UK. Presenting features include meconium ileus, recurrent respiratory infection, failure to thrive, loose stools, steatorrhoea and malabsorption. Other associated features include rectal prolapse, short stature, delayed puberty, diabetes mellitus, chronic sinusitis and nasal polyps.

3.19 A, B, D, E

3.20 A, B, D

Secondary prevention aims to prevent injury should the 'accident' happen, whereas primary prevention is aimed at preventing the 'accident' from happening and includes speed limits, stair gates, teaching road safety and child-proof catches on cupboards. Examples of secondary prevention include cycling helmets, seat belts, smoke alarms and fire extinguishers kept in the house. Note that blister packs for prescription drugs merely limit the number of tablets that a child can get at in a given time and are therefore a form of secondary prevention, whereas child-resistant lids are a form of primary prevention because they prevent the child from reaching the drug. Tertiary prevention aims to limit the impact of an injury once the 'accident' has happened and includes teaching parents first aid skills and providing good access to the emergency services.

3.21 A, B, C, D

Features of congenital rubella syndrome include deafness, eye defects (microphthalmia, cataract, retinopathy and glaucoma), cardiac defects (PDA, ASD and pulmonary stenosis), cerebral palsy, microcephaly, learning disability and osteitis. Saddle nose is a feature of congenital syphilis.

3.22 A, D

Congenital heart disease (CHD) has an incidence of 8 per 1000 live births with VSD being the most common. Acyanotic lesions (eg VSD, ASD, PDA and pulmonary stenosis) are approximately three times more common than cyanotic lesions (eg transposition of the great arteries [TGA] and Fallot's tetralogy) and generally have a better prognosis. Down's syndrome is associated with an increased incidence of VSD and ASD. Other risk factors for CHD include maternal drug and alcohol abuse, maternal diabetes, maternal infection (eg rubella), a positive family history and Turner's syndrome (eg coarctation). Indometacin is a prostaglandin synthase inhibitor and may lead to premature closure of the ductus. In TGA, intravenous prostaglandin E is given to keep the ductus open until urgent catheterisation can be carried out. Definitive surgery is postponed until the infant is aged about 9–12 months.

3.23 C, D, E

Short-term fostering is usually at an age of less than 6 months; if a longer placement is required adoption should be considered. Long-term fostering is preferred for older children, whereas adoption is more appropriate for younger children. Fostering is more likely to be successful if there are children of a similar age in the placement family. There is usually a limit of three foster children per family; however, more may be fostered if they are all siblings. All children in long-term foster care require a 6-monthly medical examination and the GP has a vital role in coordinating services and ensuring continuing medical care.

3.24 B

Aerosol inhalers are appropriate for children aged over 10 years; however, if their technique is poor, a spacer device, which allows inhaled drugs to be given adequately at any age, may be appropriate. A plastic coffee cup makes an adequate (and cheap), homemade, 'back-up' spacer device simply by making a small hole in the base for the inhaler and placing the rim firmly over the child's mouth and nose, while the metered dose is given. Dry powder inhalers are suitable for a child aged over 5 years and oral salbutamol syrup is often prescribed in primary care for the treatment of infants and toddlers, although an inhaler plus spacer device may be more beneficial.

answers

3.25 B, C, D

SIDS is defined as death of an infant or young child that is unexpected by history and in whom a thorough postmortem examination fails to reveal an adequate explanation. The incidence varies worldwide with marked seasonal variation (increases in winter months) and is the leading cause of death in infants ages over 1 week. Risk factors include male sex, multiple births, low-birthweight babies, associated respiratory infection, bottle-feeding, social classes IV and V, and the prone sleeping position (the supine position helps reduce the risk). A history of a sibling dying of SIDS increases the risk 10-fold, whereas maternal substance abuse increases the risk 30-fold. Management involves support and reassuring the parents that they are not to blame. The need for a postmortem examination should be explained and, if a twin, the sibling should be investigated and observed. The GP should visit the same day and follow up regularly over the next few weeks because, once the acute shock is over, depression may ensue.

3.26 A, B, C

Of children with cystic fibrosis 95% have pancreatic insufficiency that results in steatorrhoea and fat-soluble vitamin (A, D, E and K) deficiency that needs supplementation. Consequently, children often have excellent appetites after treatment and undiagnosed, non-compliant or unwell children are often anorectic. The investigation of choice is the sweat test – to confirm the diagnosis three tests should be abnormal (ie sweat sodium > 70 mmol/L). Cystic fibrosis is a disorder of white individuals, having a lower incidence in African–Caribbean individuals, and is very rare in Chinese individuals. Cystic fibrosis causes male infertility but not impotence.

3.27 C, D

Routine screening of all children for VUR does not fulfil the criteria of Wilson and Jungner for cost-effectiveness. There is a significant chance of VUR occurring in younger children with a UTI, especially if aged under 1 year, when a micturating cystourethrogram (MCUG) with other renal imaging is usually indicated. Investigations in children aged over 2 years are much less likely to reveal important abnormalities and, if invasive or involve ionising radiation, are indicated only selectively. Reflux nephropathy is an important cause of renal hypertension and chronic renal failure in childhood. An MCUG is the investigation of choice for diagnosis. VUR is graded as follows:

- Grade I: reflux into lower end of ureter without dilatation

- Grade II: urine refluxes into the kidney on micturition only

- Grade III: reflux enters kidney during both bladder filling and voiding

- Grade IV: reflux with dilatation of the ureter or renal pelvis.

Management of grade IV VUR is debatable and should be referred for a urological opinion. Conservative medical management may be all that is required; however, surgical re-implantation of the ureters is an option.

3.28 B, C, D

In spastic diplegia, the legs are more severely affected than the arms; in spastic hemiplegia there is asymmetrical tone and reduced movements on the affected side (arm relatively weaker than the leg) with the limbs on the affected side being smaller, colder and spastic, although almost all children are usually walking by school age. Spastic hemiplegia may result from an infarct of the cortex or internal capsule and only about 30% have an IQ < 70.

answers

3.29 A, C, D, E

There may be general signs of sexual abuse (eg superficial injuries, recurrent UTI), perineal signs (eg soreness, vaginal discharge) and behavioural signs (eg sexualised behaviour, depression, bedwetting, drug dependence). Chlamydial infection and genital warts are the common sexually transmitted infections (STIs) in child sex abuse. HIV infection in children is generally through vertical transmission; however, it may occur through sexual abuse. Anal fissures, skin tags, reflex dilatation and perianal bruising also rouse suspicion of, but are not pathognomonic for, sexual abuse.

3.30 B, C, E

Acute renal failure (ARF) is a sudden disturbance of renal function resulting in decreased urine output with rising serum urea and creatinine. There are three main causes of ARF:

1. Prerenal: caused by hypovolaemia (eg burns) or hypotension (eg septicaemia)

2. Renal, eg haemolytic uraemic syndrome, acute glomerulonephritis and nephrotoxins (ie gentamicin)

3. Postrenal: caused by congenital (eg urethral valves) or acquired (eg renal calculi) obstructive uropathy.

Management involves resuscitation, fluid restriction, correction of electrolytes, intravenous antibiotics if septic, a high-calorie/low-protein diet (total parenteral nutrition [TPN] may be necessary) and possibly dialysis. Indications for dialysis include a diuretic-resistant hypervolaemia with hypertension and pulmonary oedema, a plasma urea > 54 mmol/L, hyperkalaemia, metabolic acidosis or a dialysable nephrotoxin. ARF may be complicated by convulsions and tetany, which are secondary to the associated hypocalcaemia and hypomagnesaemia.

3.31 B, D, E

The BTS guidelines define severe acute asthma as: too breathless to talk; too breathless to feed; respiration > 50 breaths/min; pulse > 140 beats/min; and PEFR < 50% predicted or best. Life-threatening features are defined as: PEFR < 33% predicted or best; cyanosis, a silent chest, or poor respiratory effort; fatigue or exhaustion; and agitation or decreased level of consciousness. Children with severe attacks may not appear distressed and assessment in young children may be difficult. Therefore, the presence of any of the above features should alert the doctor.

3.32 A, C, D, E

Infantile colic characteristically presents with paroxysmal crying of the infant and 'pulling up' of the legs; infrequently it lasts beyond 3 months of age. Colic is not a diagnosis of exclusion, although it is important to consider serious pathology when seeing a child with colic. Colic should be viewed as a symptom that has some known causes (eg cows' milk protein intolerance), but often no cause can be found. Although there is no clinically effective treatment, the child may require social admission to hospital to break the cycle of stressed mother and crying baby.

3.33 A, B, C, E

UTIs are more common in boys in the first month of life and become more common in girls from about 6 months. *E. coli* is responsible for about 80% of cases. Other causative organisms include *Klebsiella* spp., *Streptomyces albus* and *Proteus* spp. In neonates most UTIs are haematogenous in origin, whereas in older infants and children infection generally ascends from the native bowel flora. About 35% of all children presenting with a UTI have VUR, with 45% of these having some structural or functional abnormality of their urinary tract (90% if < 2 years and 60% if < 5 years). The diagnosis of VUR is most important in the under-2s because this is the age group most likely to develop reflux nephropathy. In older age groups, there is a move away from investigating for VUR because the clinical sequelae are less clear cut. Significant bacteriuria from a normal midstream urine (MSU) or clean catch has > 105 CFU of bacteria/mL; however, a suprapubic aspirate requires > 103 CFU/mL only.

answers

3.34 A, B, C, D, E

Primary generalised tonic–clonic epilepsy has no known cause and typically presents after age 5 years. There is usually no aura, although these auras do occur in partial seizures with secondary generalised seizures. Features include an initial tonic spasm associated with collapse, loss of consciousness and cyanosis lasting more than 60 s. This is usually followed by clonic spasms with/without incontinence and tongue biting lasting more than 3 min. The ensuing post-ictal phase or coma gradually resolves over several minutes to hours with headache, drowsiness, confusion and myalgia. Complications include status epilepticus, which is a fit (or consecutive fits without complete recovery between) lasting more than 30 min. The EEG may be normal between seizures or show bursts of spike waves. During the tonic phase, diffuse runs of spike waves occur, with slow waves alternating with spike waves in the clonic phase. First-line treatment is carbamazepine or valproate, with 70% of patients being fit free on monotherapy alone. Other antiepileptic drugs include lamotrigine, with newer drugs such as topiramate and levetiracetam being used more often and phenytoin and phenobarbital being used less often. After 15 years, 80% will remain in remission off treatment altogether.

3.35 B, C, D, E

NAI should be suspected when there is a delay in presentation of the child with an inadequate or inconsistent explanation of the symptoms or lesions. An unusual parental attitude, such as overprotection or alternatively appearing unconcerned, should also cause concern. Accidental skull fractures tend to be single, linear, narrow and parietal with rarely any associated intracranial injury. A depressed skull fracture is therefore highly suspicious, as is a fractured tibia in a non-ambulant child aged 6 months. It is difficult for an infant to develop black eyes except through a punching injury, so unilateral, and particularly bilateral, black eyes are suggestive of abuse.

Answers to Extending Matching Questions

3.36 Respiratory distress in the newborn

1   I – Surfactant deficient lung disease (hyaline membrane disease)

Although all of the options are possible, it is the most likely one from the information given. Pulmonary hypoplasia and persistent pulmonary hypertension of the newborn are also possible but the most common cause of respiratory distress syndrome (RDS) at birth at 24 weeks' gestation is hyaline membrane disease (HMD).

2   H – Pulmonary hypoplasia

As the fetal lungs require amniotic fluid to develop properly, rupture of the membranes at 16 weeks will lead to oligohydramnios and subsequent pulmonary hypoplasia. Erythromycin reduces the incidence of congenital pneumonia. HMD is less likely at 33 weeks' gestation.

3   J – Transient tachypnoea of the newborn

Transient tachypnoea of the newborn is the most likely diagnosis because caesarean sections don't provide stimulation for absorption of lung fluid. This would be the most likely diagnosis if there were an uncomplicated antenatal course.

answers

3.37 Genetic diseases

1   A – Autosomal dominant

Achondroplasia is an autosomal dominant condition; however, 90% of occurrences are as a result of a new mutation.

2   C – Autosomal recessive

Sickle cell disease is a good example of an autosomal recessive inherited condition. The chance of inheritance of the disease (HbSS) is one in four if both parents are heterozygotes (HbSs). The prevalence of the gene in the population is increased because the heterozygote form (sickle cell trait) provides resistance to malaria in endemic countries.

3   J – X-linked recessive

Duchenne muscular dystrophy occurs in 1 in 3000 live male births. There is a significant new mutation rate of 30%. The underlying abnormality is a decreased production of dystrophin. Presentation is usually in early childhood, and there may be a history of delay in walking and a tendency to fall. Difficulty in getting up from a sitting position can be demonstrated (Gower's sign). Hip flexion contractures and calf hypertrophy lead to toe walking. Of those affected 90% are wheel-chair bound by puberty and 30% have some learning disability.

3.38 Blood disorders

1   E – G6PDH deficiency

G6PDH deficiency is more common in people of Mediterranean origin (up to 35%). Haemolysis can be triggered by a number of factors (favism, antimalarials, sulphonamides, etc) – in this case probably nitrofurantoin, sometimes given for UTIs. The picture is of a haemolytic anaemia: there is a very good reticulocyte response showing that bone marrow production is good. Thalassaemia is unlikely because this presented as an acute problem.

2   H – Immune-mediated thrombocytopenia purpura

This is a typical picture of immune-mediated thrombocytopenia purpura. The low platelet count is a result of peripheral destruction of platelets, not failure of production (megakaryocytes are precursors of platelets in the bone marrow).

3   G – Henoch–Schönlein purpura

The distribution of the rash is consistent with Henoch–Schönlein purpura. In a well child, with normal platelets and clotting, meningococcal septicaemia is less likely; however, it should always be considered.

3.39 Infant nutrition

1   E – 1 year

Pasta contains gluten, which should be avoided until 1 year of age.

2   B – 4 months

Baby rice is a good food to start weaning. Weaning should start at 4–6 months (although the WHO recommends exclusive breast-feeding until 6 months of age).

3   C – 7 months

answers

3.40 Systemic diseases

1   C – Kawasaki's disease

The major criteria of Kawasaki's disease are: cervical lymphadenopathy (> 2 cm), non-purulent conjunctivitis, mucositis, high spiking fever for > 5 days, polymorphous rash/extremity change.

2   B – Dermatomyositis

The age of the girl makes some diagnoses more likely than others (eg dermatomyositis, SLE). However, the rash affecting the eyelids is characteristic of dermatomyositis, along with the raised CK. The pain in the knees and legs is caused by the myositis and not an arthritis as such.

3   E – Pauciarticular juvenile idiopathic arthritis

Double-stranded DNA (dsDNA) negative makes SLE unlikely; ASOT negative renders rheumatic fever unlikely. The clinical picture fits with that of juvenile idiopathic arthritis (previously called juvenile chronic arthritis). This is pauciarticular because it involves four or less joints. ANA positive means that there is a high risk of iridocyclitis and the patient must be screened for this.

3.41 Syndromes

1   G – Pierre Robin syndrome

These are typical features for Pierre Robin syndrome. The mandibular hypoplasia causes a degree of glossoptosis (tongue obstructing airway posteriorly). These infants should be nursed prone and may often require a nasopharyngeal airway to be used until the face/jaw has grown sufficiently. In the absence of associated syndromes/features, intelligence is normal.

2   E – Noonan syndrome

Noonan syndrome has a similar phenotype to Turner's syndrome, but can occur in both sexes. There is often a degree of learning difficulties. Noonan syndrome has an association with right-sided cardiac defects (especially pulmonary stenosis).

3   D – Fragile X syndrome

In any child with marked behavioural or learning difficulties, if no other cause is obvious, fragile X syndrome should always be considered. Fragile X is the second most common genetic cause (trinucleotide repeat sequences on the X chromosome) for learning difficulties in males (Down's syndrome being the most common). Phenotypically, children with fragile X syndrome have large ears, long noses and high foreheads. Testicular volume is markedly increased.

answers

3.42 Immunisations

1   F – Palivizumab

Ex-pre-term infants with chronic lung disease are at a much higher risk from respiratory infections. RSV is a major concern for babies with chronic lung disease, leading to high rates of hospital admission, PICU admission and even mortality. The evidence for passive immunisation against RSV shows that it will not prevent infection or hospital admission with RSV bronchiolitis (in babies with chronic lung disease). However, it seems to reduce the severity of the illness, such that it reduces the need for PICU admission (NNT = 10 to prevent 1 PICU admission.) There is some debate about whether this is cost-effective. Most neonatal ICUs will arrange the immunisation of babies with chronic lung disease.

2   E – Influenza vaccine

A child receiving chemotherapy for AML will be significantly immunosuppressed. If such a child has siblings, it is important that they are immunised against influenza, which can be devastating to an immunosuppressed child. Previously a sibling would have received inactivated polio rather than live oral polio vaccine; however, since the change to the universal schedule (where all polio is inactivated) this is no longer a consideration.

3   J – Unconjugated pneumococcal vaccine

This child may or may not have been part of the conjugated pneumococcal vaccine catch-up programme; however, as she is over 2 years old, it is important that she receive the unconjugated vaccine. At this age she will be able to make a good antibody response to the vaccine and the unconjugated vaccine protects against 30–40 pneumococcal serotypes (compared with 7 serotypes for the conjugated vaccine).

3.43 Drugs

1   E – Per os azithromycin

This 12-year-old has presented with a clinical chest infection but has no signs of acute respiratory distress. A macrolide is a very reasonable choice in this situation because it will cover common pathogens such as pneumococci but also mycoplasmas, which must be considered in a child of this age. Azithromycin is a newer macrolide that is given once a day for 3 days; this low dosing regimen is argued to improve compliance.

2   A – Intravenous aciclovir

In any child with headache and a fever, meningitis/encephalitis should be considered. If the child has a seizure, the index of suspicion is much higher. Temporal lobe changes are classically seen on CT in herpes encephalitis. Intravenous aciclovir is the therapy of choice for herpes encephalitis. In a real-life scenario, this child would also have received a broad-spectrum antibiotic (eg intravenous cefotaxime) to cover bacterial causes.

3   H – Intravenous co-amoxiclav

The two most likely pathogens in this situation are *S. aureus* and *Streptococcus* spp. As the child is displaying systemic symptoms and the infection is in more than two areas, it would be reasonable to treat with a broad-spectrum antibiotic that covers both pathogens. Augmentin would be appropriate in this case. Intravenous flucloxacillin alone is not sufficient unless combined with benzylpenicillin.

Best of Five Answers

3.44 B

'The most important to exclude': intussusception is the only one that is potentially life threatening. The others are, of course, possible diagnoses but not immediately life threatening.

3.45 C

These symptoms are classic of croup. The most common cause is parainfluenza 3.

3.46 C

Although all of the answers would cause the listed symptoms, pyloric stenosis, jejunal stenosis and gastroenteritis would be very unlikely in a thriving child. The daily volume of feed is quite substantial (1200 mL) and in a 5 kg baby would work out to 240 mL/kg per day! Approximately 150 mL/kg per day is a rough guide to a baby's milk requirement.

3.47 D

Increase in testicular volume is the first sign of puberty in boys (from 10 years). Voice change occurs at around 14 years. Peak height velocity is when testicular volume reaches 10 mL (pubic hair stage 4). There is a wide range in times of onset of the stages in individuals.

(A good reference for sequence of development is Marshall WA, Tanner, JM (1970) Variations in the pattern of pubertal changes in boys. *Archives of Diseases in Childhood* **45**:13–23.)

3.48 D

In a child with no respiratory distress there is no need to admit unless oral antibiotics cannot be tolerated. The BTS guidelines for community-acquired pneumonia in children suggest the use of a macrolide antibiotic as a first line in the over-5s if *Mycoplasma* sp. is a possible causative organism. If, however, there are features that would suggest pneumococcal chest infection (focal consolidation/signs), then amoxicillin is the suggested first-line treatment.

3.49 A

Stridor indicates an upper airway problem. Croup is less likely in an unwell child, especially if there has been a preceding tonsillitis. Epiglottitis would be surprising in a child immunised with Hib, but it is recognised. Bacterial tracheitis is indeed a possibility but, with a preceding tonsillitis, a retropharyngeal abscess is more likely.

3.50 C

Gillick competence is important to understand. Lord Fraser held that a girl under 16 years of age could be prescribed the oral contraceptive pill (OCP) if the following criteria could be met:

1. The girl can understand, retain and make informed decisions based on the information given to her.

2. That, despite discussion, she will definitely not involve her parents.

3. If she is going to have sexual intercourse whether or not the OCP is prescribed.

4. If the OCP is NOT prescribed, it will be detrimental to her health.

5. If it is in her best interests.

There is now a move away from calling these criteria 'Gillick competence' to 'Fraser competent'.

3.51 B

Typical features of a febrile convulsion are: age 6 months to 6 years and febrile (or rising temperature) at time of convulsion. Generalised tonic–clonic seizures last up to 10 min with a post-ictal phase afterwards. The eyes rolling back and incontinence are often seen. Focal features of secondarily generalised seizures are sometimes seen in febrile convulsions but are not typical. A rapid recovery is uncharacteristic of a generalised tonic–clonic seizure – whether febrile or afebrile. The duration of the seizures in D and E means that these are not typical. Prolonged seizures (25 min) and repeated seizures are not typical febrile seizures.

answers

3.52 C

Discussion of potential morbidity and mortality with parents in threatened premature labour is difficult but very important. If there is a threatened delivery at 23 weeks' gestation it is important to discuss with the parents the possibility of not resuscitating if the condition of the baby is poor or the gestation looks to be earlier, because the outcome is likely to be very poor. It is useful to give parents morbidity and mortality figures – either national figures from the EPICURE study (*Pediatrics 2000*;**106**:659–71) or, preferably, the figures for your own unit.

3.53 A

- Six-word vocabulary: by 2 years
- > 100-word vocabulary: 2 years
- Two- to three-word phrases: by 25 months
- Tuneful babbling: by 8 months
- Sing nursery rhymes: by 3 years.

3.54 E

Grading of intraventricular haemorrhage is as follows:

- Grade 1: ependymal (germinal matrix)
- Grade 2: intraventricular without ventricular dilatation
- Grade 3: intraventricular with ventricular dilatation
- Grade 4: parenchymal.

Prognosis depends on grade of bleed: grades 1 and 2 have a good prognosis with no long-term effects. In grade 3 there may be possible impairment on the contralateral side, depending on the degree of progression of dilatation, and in grade 4 there is likely to be motor impairment on the contralateral side.

3.55 E

Gynaecomastia is not uncommon in puberty in boys and resolves spontaneously. Bullying is not acceptable and schools have very good anti-bullying policies. Surgical reduction is a last resort in gynaecomastia that doesn't resolve. Psychological support may be useful but will not stop the bullying itself.

3.56 C

Although it is within the remit of the CCDC – part of the public health department – to contact, trace and treat the necessary family members, it is good practice to liaise with them and treat the contacts at risk. This is easier for the acute clinicians to do because the contacts (usually family members) are often with the unwell child.

3.57 E

APLS (*Advanced Paediatric Life Support* – see answer to Question 2.41, page 174) recommendations indicate that tibial interosseus needle insertion is a quick and easy method of securing venous access in an arrested child. The other methods are satisfactory but, in a collapsed child, may be difficult and time-consuming to insert.

3.58 C

The most likely diagnosis is a torted cyst of Morgagni (an embryonic remnant on the poles of the testes). However, the most important diagnosis to exclude is testicular torsion and so most will undergo surgical exploration. Mumps orchitis is rare now because of MMR. Infertility secondary to mumps orchitis is rare (< 1%).

3.59 C

The only medical indication for circumcision is balanitis xeroderma obliterans (BXO). A non-retractile foreskin is not uncommon until puberty. The adhesions may be released with some weak steroid cream. Ballooning of the foreskin is not a problem in itself.

3.60 B

Carbamazepine is a good first-line anticonvulsant. Plasma levels are easily monitored if control is not achieved. Carbamazepine is not as hepatotoxic as sodium valproate, and is less cardiotoxic than phenytoin (which also has zero-order kinetics, making dose titration difficult). Diazepam as needed is not a realistic treatment because the aim is to prevent seizures – not to treat them when they happen.

3.61 A

Treatment of eczema can be problematic. It is worthwhile giving parents advice about simple, everyday measures that can improve the eczema: using non-biological washing powder; wearing cotton clothes as opposed to artificial fibres; and not using soaps or shampoos. Use of a bath oil (eg Oilatum) is beneficial and aqueous cream can be used as 'soap' to good effect. Regular emollient use is important; however, parents can find using very greasy products hard work because it involves a lot of washing of clothes. The aim is to keep the skin from feeling dry at any time of day. Sedating with older types of antihistamines at night does not help to reduce itching, but used occasionally in large doses provides a sedative effect that may improve sleep. Once all these measures are in use, but the eczema is still not controlled, escalation of treatment would be appropriate. There is no evidence for the benefit of topical antibiotics.

3.62 B

In an infant who has had a confirmed UTI and pelvicalyceal dilatation on ultrasonography, an MCUG is important to look for VUR. If present, VUR greatly increases the risk for renal scarring when associated with UTIs and so prophylactic antibiotics are important to try to prevent repeat UTIs.

answers

3.63 C

This patient has an abscess that has developed secondary to caries in her lower left 'E'. She has lymphadenitis secondary to this and, as the swelling is fluctuant, there is probably an abscess there. If there is a large (> 1 cm) abscess present, the treatment is incision and drainage with postoperative antibiotics. Antibiotics as a first line may reduce the infection, but will not treat it completely if the abscess is large. In the case of a small periodental/dental abscess, a course of oral antibiotics may treat the abscess, but advice to see a GDP should be reinforced.

3.64 C

The most practical and reliable device to deliver inhaled medication to a 5-year-old is a spacing device, which can also be used for preventive measures and is particularly effective as a relief medication. Nebulisers are relatively impractical, less portable, take longer to deliver each dose and expensive. Most 5-year-olds are usually unable to use a dry powder device very reliably and even less so MDIs. Oral leukotriene antagonists are not first-line therapy in asthma prevention.

3.65 D

This 7-year-old with cerebral palsy has 'dystonic' movements associated with feeding, which also appear to exacerbate with chest infections. These have not been noted at other times and specifically no intention tremor or incoordination has been noted. The constellation of symptoms is compatible with severe gastro-oesophageal reflux and oesophagitis, which can lead to dystonic movements as a result of the extreme discomfort, especially at and after meals. The reflux can be the cause of recurrent chestiness and wheeze, which may present as or exacerbate pre-existing asthma. The diagnosis of epilepsy needs to be revised in the absence of a compatible clinical picture, absence of response to antiepileptic drugs and presence of normal EEGs.

3.66 E

An ECG may show abnormalities such as right ventricular hypertrophy, but this will not explain the week-long history of symptoms. A raised ASOT will demonstrate past streptococcal infection, but the rash is not that of rheumatic fever, ie erythema marginatum. The most likely diagnosis, which needs to be confirmed, is of infective endocarditis; this needs to be proved by at least three blood cultures taken before antibiotic treatment is started. An echocardiogram may show vegetations if present, but if absent does not exclude the diagnosis.

3.67 E

Soaps and shampoos are irritant to the middle ear, and the soap in the water theoretically allows the liquid to pass more easily through the hole in the grommet itself. As daily washing is the most common of these activities, it follows that this is the most important advice. Swimming in swimming pools is permitted although diving and underwater swimming should be discouraged. Sea water is more likely to cause infection than chlorinated pool water, but swimming may be allowed if the ears are appropriately plugged. There should not be any hearing loss with grommets, and grommets may ease any pressure equalisation problems on aeroplane flights. There is little evidence base to this and much variation in advice from ENT surgeons re management, but the above is based on the Prodigy clinical knowledge summaries.

3.68 E

Of the management options listed for this girl with encopresis, a referral to the CAMHS team is the most appropriate. She is already taking mild laxatives with good effect, with little to suggest significant constipation because she passes normal stools regularly, although not in the toilet. A Social Services referral may be indicated at some time, but is mainly indicated if there are specific child protection concerns. Behavioural programmes may well be helpful, but not using negative rewards which may well be counterproductive and be experienced as punishment.

Multiple Choice Answers

4.1 A, D, E

Antiepileptics taken antenatally increase the incidence of cleft lip and palate. Cleft lip should be repaired at 3 months, but a cleft palate repair should be done between 6 months and 1 year. If surgery is performed during this time and the help of a speech and language therapist enlisted, speech has about a 75% chance of developing normally. Cleft palate may cause hearing loss as a result of the increased incidence of otitis media with effusion. Admission to an SCBU should be avoided because this can hinder bonding. Special teats are available to use before surgical repair if feeding is problematic.

4.2 B, E

The prevalence of asthma is increased in males, a personal or first-degree family history of atopy and among urban dwellers. Maternal smoking during pregnancy or passive smoking postnatally is also associated with an increased prevalence. Forceps delivery bears no relationship to the risk of developing asthma, although a low birthweight is relevant.

4.3   A, D, E

Infantile spasms are rare with usual onset between 4 and 9 months. The infants characteristically present with 'jack-knife' or 'salaam' attacks, which involve sudden flexion of the trunk, head and arms. These spasms typically last only a second but can recur several times a minute ('drop attacks' are characteristic of myoclonic astatic epilepsy). The inter-ictal EEG shows hypsarrhythmia in 66% and 70% will have localised or diffuse brain lesions on CT (tuberous sclerosis, brain malformations and chronic trauma), whereas 30% have no identifiable cause. The children with brain damage are refractory to treatment and develop psychomotor disabilities by age 5 years, whereas cryptogenic cases respond better to treatment – seizures settle by 5 years and 50% develop a normal IQ. First-line treatment is prednisolone or ACTH for 3 months, followed by benzodiazepines or valproate.

4.4   B, D

No vaccine is contraindicated in cerebral palsy and full immunisation should be encouraged. Feeding difficulties occur as a result of hypertonia and problems arise because of the persistence of primitive reflexes (eg Moro's reflex, the grasp reflex and the asymmetrical tonic neonatal reflex).

4.5   A, B, C

There are certain common factors that predispose to child abuse, including parental factors, such as coming from a broken home, and possibly being abused themselves and thus lacking a suitable role model on which to base good parenting skills. The parent may have a personality disorder or psychiatric illness. Risk factors associated with the child include prematurity, especially if the child was admitted to a SCBU. The ensuing maternal separation results in a threefold risk of abuse. Other features are children from unwanted pregnancies or those with a chronic illness or behavioural problems. The great majority of abused children are aged under 4 years. Social factors are also an issue; any family crisis (eg bereavement, unemployment) increases the risk of abuse. Drug/alcohol dependence, poor housing, stepchildren, maternal exhaustion and social isolation are also all features. An extended family nearby lessens the risk.

4.6   A, D, E

Pica is defined as the 'eating of things that are not food'. It is likely to be associated with other signs of disturbed behaviour or a decreased IQ. If disciplinary approaches are unsuccessful, a community paediatric referral may be appropriate to assess any developmental delay. It is associated with iron deficiency anaemia, although it is not fully understood how or why, but may respond to a short course of iron supplements. The 'mouthing' of objects seen at 8 months is a normal transient developmental phase. However, if this persists beyond 2 years of age it is likely to be associated with some developmental problem.

4.7   B, C, D, E

ADD is the term applied to unusually overactive children with accompanying lack of concentration, impulsiveness and emotional immaturity; boys are affected more than girls in a ratio of 5:1. Various associations include lead poisoning, drugs (eg phenobarbital, phenytoin and theophylline) and possibly food additives (eg tartrazine [E102], sunset yellow [E110], carmoisine [E122] and amaranth). Other foods that may exacerbate hyperactivity in some children include cows' milk and wheat, although the evidence for this is weak. ADD is diagnosed more frequently in the USA. In the UK it is felt to be uncommon in isolation, but possibly occurs more frequently in association with conduct disorders or learning disability. Psychosocial assessment, which involves counselling parents and teaching simple behaviour modification techniques, is the mainstay of treatment. Medical treatment includes Ritalin (methylphenidate hydrochloride) and dietary advice may also have a role in a minority of children.

4.8 A, B, C, E

Salicylate poisoning can cause both respiratory alkalosis and metabolic acidosis. However, although respiratory alkalosis is a common finding in adults, children tend to have a more prominent metabolic acidosis. Hyperglycaemia, and hypoglycaemia, occur in salicylate poisoning. A serum salicylate level < 400 mg/L is rarely symptomatic, whereas levels > 1.2 g/L are usually lethal. The mainstay of treatment involves correcting acidosis, hypoglycaemia and dehydration with intravenous fluid replacement, while ensuring a urine output of 5–6 mL/kg per h. Urgent dialysis may be required for acute renal failure. Salicylate poisoning may also result in hypoprothrombinaemia, which can cause a coagulopathy requiring correction with vitamin K and fresh frozen plasma (FFP).

4.9 B, C, E

Tuberculin testing traditionally involves an injection into the flexor surface of the left forearm. The Heaf test is no longer available. The Mantoux test is read at 48–72 h (but up to 96 h). A positive result occurs when the area of induration is > 5 mm. Note that the area of 'flare' is irrelevant. Good practice is not to 'grade' the response; rather write down the actual measurement of induration. A good guide to the Mantoux test can be found at www.immunisation. nhs.uk/files/mantouxtest.pdf.

4.10 A, C, D, E

Sickle cell anaemia is an autosomal recessive condition that results from synthesis of an abnormal Hb chain (HbS). It is common among black people with 40% of black Africans and 10% of British African–Caribbean individuals carrying HbS. It can be diagnosed by fetal blood sampling at around 18/40 or earlier by fetal DNA analysis of cells from the amniotic fluid or trophoblast biopsy.

Heterozygotes (sickle cell trait) are usually asymptomatic unless severely hypoxic, and typically have a normal haemoglobin and blood film. Homozygotes (sickle cell disease), however, present with acute haemolysis and frequent painful sickling crises of mainly the fingers and toes from the age of about 6 months, and larger joints from 3–4 years. Their haemoglobin is usually around 6–8 g/dL and their blood films typically show hypochromia, target cells, Howell–Jolly bodies and occasional sickle cells. The associated chronic haemolytic anaemia results in an increased incidence of pigment gallstones, leading to biliary colic.

Management involves supportive measures using fluids, oxygen and analgesia. Antibiotics, blood or even exchange transfusion may also be necessary acutely. Splenectomy should be considered for hypersplenism or recurrent sequestration crises and should always be covered with pneumococcal immunisation with or without prophylactic penicillin.

4.11 A, C, D

Reye syndrome is acute encephalopathy with fatty degeneration of the liver, kidneys and pancreas, resulting in vomiting, delirium, fits and coma. Other features include hepatomegaly, hypoglycaemia, cerebral oedema and hyperammonaemia. The aetiology is unclear, but viral illness and aspirin exposure have been postulated as precipitating risk factors. Indeed there has been a steady decline in incidence since 1986 when aspirin was withdrawn from routine use in young children. It usually presents before the age of 2 years after a prodromal illness and is associated with a high mortality. The transaminases are typically elevated, but bilirubin is usually normal. Treatment involves general supportive measures and reduction of any raised intracranial pressures, with normalisation of the $Paco_2$ and intravenous mannitol. Complications include renal failure, gastrointestinal bleeding and pancreatitis, and should be managed accordingly.

4.12 C, E

The characteristic features of Fallot's tetralogy are a ventricular septal defect, pulmonary stenosis, an overriding aorta and ventricular hypertrophy resulting in a right-to-left shunt. Fallot's tetralogy and TGA are the two leading causes of cyanotic congenital heart disease. In Fallot's tetralogy, central cyanosis occurs with infundibular spasm, which is relieved by propranolol. There is no murmur associated with the VSD; however, the pulmonary stenosis typically results in an ejection systolic murmur heard best over the pulmonary area. The characteristic chest radiological appearance of Fallot's tetralogy is a 'boot-shaped' cardiac shadow, whereas the 'egg on its side' is more typical of TGA.

4.13 A

Vasoconstriction of the ophthalmic artery occurs in simple migraine, resulting in a transient visual aura, scintillating scotoma, zigzag lines (fortification phenomenon), visual field defects and micropsia. Strabismus, diplopia and nystagmus are all signs of possible intracranial pathology. Papilloedema is a sign of raised intracranial pressure that indicates more serious intracranial pathology.

4.14 A, B, C

Down's syndrome is the leading cause of severe learning difficulties. It affects about 1 in 660 births. Trisomy 21 is responsible for 90% of cases and has a recurrence risk of about 1%. The incidence increases with maternal age, with a woman of 40 years having a 1 in 40 risk. Typical features include developmental delay with an IQ between 20 and 75. They have a characteristic appearance of upslanting eyes with wide epicanthic folds, a small nose with a low bridge, a small mouth with a protruding tongue, a single palmar crease and general hypotonia/joint laxity. A cardiac lesion, particularly a PDA or ASD, is present in 40%. Other common disorders include duodenal atresia, thyroid disease and leukaemia.

4.15 B, C, D, E

Both haemophilia A and B are X-linked disorders and result from deficient factor VIII coagulation. In both conditions the intrinsic clotting pathway is affected, resulting in a prolonged activated thromboplastin ratio (APTR). The prothrombin time measures the extrinsic pathway and is therefore normal. Haemophilia presents with an increased risk of haemorrhage into soft tissue, resulting in bruising and recurrent haemarthroses (leading to progressive joint destruction) after surgery or dental extraction, rendering prophylactic dental care essential. Management of acute bleeds requires the prompt administration of factor VIII concentrate (or cryoprecipitate/FFP). Aspirin and intramuscular injections are strongly contraindicated and a haematological opinion should be sought before any surgical procedure.

4.16 A, B

In the UK, cows' milk protein intolerance is the most common cause of chronic diarrhoea in infants aged under 1 year. Other common causes include constipation with overflow, after gastroenteritis (eg lactose intolerance), infections (eg *Salmonella, Giardia* spp.) and toddler diarrhoea, which is characterised by recognisable food in the stool of a thriving child (peas-and-carrots syndrome). Coeliac disease is caused by sensitivity to gluten in wheat and rye, which results in the characteristic jejunal villous atrophy seen at biopsy, leading to malabsorption. However, this is not diagnostic, because similar appearances may be found with gastroenteritis and cows' milk intolerance. Diagnosis is made initially by the presence of IgA anti-transglutaminase antibodies, followed by the characteristic changes on biopsy. It is clinically confirmed by remission within weeks of starting a gluten-free diet and subsequent reduction of the circulating IgA-specific antibodies. It has an incidence of about 1 in 2000 and tends to run in families, with girls being more commonly affected. It usually presents at between 9 months and 3 years with failure to thrive and frequent loose stools, although mild cases may remain undiagnosed into adulthood. Diffuse inflammation and ulceration of the colon characterise ulcerative colitis; it is rare in childhood and not inherited in a mendelian fashion.

4.17 A, B, D, E

Appendicitis is rare in the under-5s, but almost 90% of cases present with perforation, demonstrating the difficulty in diagnosis. Problems may be a result of the child's ineloquent history and, because of its rarity, it is not considered initially. In addition it may be difficult to localise pain in a small abdomen. Retrocaecal appendicitis may not cause any localising signs (per rectum examination reveals tenderness anteriorly) or the child may present with urinary symptoms/signs if a pelvic appendix is inflamed. A useful sign is the child's ability to 'hop' or 'jump' because peritonitis is excluded if this is painless, making the diagnosis of appendicitis unlikely. Differential diagnoses include mesenteric adenitis, UTI, diabetic ketoacidosis, intussusception, lower lobe pneumonia and infectious hepatitis.

4.18 A, B

The health visitor relieves the midwife of responsibility at 10 days post delivery and is subsequently responsible for child health surveillance in all children up to age 5 years. They are informed of every child under 5 who attends A&E and A&E are obliged to contact the health visitor of any child who needs appropriate follow-up. Health visitors also supervise the running of immunisation clinics; however, social workers are responsible for children in care.

4.19 A, B, E

Anorexia nervosa occurs predominantly among teenage girls, affecting 1 in 250 between the ages of 15 and 18 years, although boys represent up to 5% of cases. Features include persistent refusal to eat, leading to potentially dangerous weight loss, intense fear of becoming obese, disturbed perception of body image and primary or secondary amenorrhoea as a result of endocrine disturbance (low luteinising hormone [LH], follicle-stimulating hormone [FSH] and oestrogen). Note that amenorrhoea before weight loss should arouse suspicion of hypothalamic dysfunction.

Symptoms may include excessive exercise, laxative/diuretic abuse and induction of vomiting which may result in hypokalaemia. Other physical complications include sensitivity to cold, constipation, faints, lethargy, hypotension and hypoglycaemia. The aetiology is multifactorial with family dynamics a key issue. Management involves gaining the patient's trust and outpatient psychotherapy for mild cases. Admission in severe cases involves treatment of medical complications, family therapy, individual psychotherapy including privileges for weight gain and occasionally drugs (eg anxiolytics, antidepressants). Depression and suicide attempts are common. About 50% remain underweight with psychological difficulties and the overall mortality rates are up to 8%.

answers

4.20 C, D, E

Neisseria gonorrhoeae may cause ophthalmia neonatorum; however, *Chlamydia* sp. is more frequently responsible. Stevens–Johnson syndrome is a systemic disorder associated with erythema multiforme ('target' lesions), fever, mouth and genital lesions, and keratitis. Orbital cellulitis presents with significant orbital oedema, limitation of ocular movements, fever and visual loss. Causes include adjacent sinusitis, bacteraemia and other local infection. Intrauterine infections that predispose to neonatal cataracts include toxoplasmosis, rubella, cytomegalovirus (CMV), herpes simplex virus and varicella-zoster virus. Other causes include autosomal inheritance and chromosomal disorders (eg Down's syndrome), metabolic disorders (eg diabetes mellitus), trauma and the use of systemic steroids. Glaucoma is rare in childhood and results from defective drainage of aqueous humour from the anterior chamber. It may be caused by primary causes such as aniridia or secondary causes such as iritis, trauma or intraocular tumour.

4.21 A

Before adoption proceeds, informed consent from both natural parents (or just the mother if unmarried) is desirable. However, it is not needed if they cannot be found, are incapable of agreeing, have abandoned or neglected the child, or have persistently ill-treated the child and are unlikely ever to be able to look after the child adequately. Applicants wanting to adopt a child must be aged 21 or more and adoption is arranged through registered agencies. The child must live with the adoptive parents for 3 months before the order is finalised, at which time all rights and responsibilities pass irreversibly to the adoptive parents. The original parents have no right of access. The adopted child takes on the nationality of the adoptive parents and has no claim to maintenance or inheritance from the original parent(s). At the age of 18 years an adopted child is entitled to his or her original birth certificate.

answers

4.22 A, B, C, E

Rickets is the inadequate mineralisation of new bone in developing bones (osteomalacia in adults). It is most commonly secondary to vitamin D deficiency (eg diet, malabsorption or lack of exposure to sunlight). Other associations include chronic renal failure and anticonvulsant therapy, because phenytoin and phenobarbital induce liver enzymes, resulting in accelerated breakdown of cholecalciferol to its inactive metabolite. Inherited causes include vitamin D-dependent (autosomal recessive) and vitamin D-resistant (X-linked dominant trait) rickets.

Clinical features include frontal bossing, kyphoscoliosis, hypotonia, swelling at the wrist and costochondral junctions ('rickety rosary'). Bow-legs (genu varum) are more usual in toddlers, whereas knock-knees (genu valgum) are typical of older children. Tetany and convulsions secondary to hypocalcaemia may occur. Treatment of nutritional rickets involves parental education and high-dose vitamin D supplements for 4–6 weeks, followed by a low dose until biochemical resolution.

4.23 A, C, D, E

4.24 A, B, D, E

Acute lymphoblastic leukaemia has a 50–75% 5-year disease-free survival rate, but approximately 10% relapse within the first year. Poor prognostic features include age < 2 years or > 10 years, a presenting WCC > 20 000/mm^3, T- or B-cell surface markers, elevated acid phosphatase in T-cell leukaemia, an anterior mediastinal mass or CNS signs at presentation. Being white is a good prognostic factor. Boys, however, have a worse prognosis, which results partly from the difference in ALL phenotype. The difference in outcomes is decreasing.

4.25 A, D

Crohn's disease is characterised by inflammation of the whole thickness of the bowel, especially the terminal ileum and proximal colon; the rectum is usually spared. The incidence has increased over the past 20–30 years and now affects about 5 per 100 000 individuals. Presenting features include failure to thrive, mouth ulcers, anorexia, abdominal pain and diarrhoea. Other non-gastrointestinal features include erythema nodosum, arthritis, digital clubbing and anaemia. Investigations include a malabsorption and infection screen, endoscopy, biopsy and barium meal, which may reveal the characteristic 'string sign', 'skip lesion' and 'rose thorn ulcers' seen in Crohn's disease.

Ulcerative colitis classically has diffuse inflammation and ulceration of the entire rectal and colonic mucosa, and is also associated with an incidence of 5 per 100 000. It typically presents around 10 years of age with intermittent episodes of abdominal pain and bloody diarrhoea. Other features include lethargy, fever, clubbing, mouth ulcers, anaemia, arthritis, short stature, erythema nodosum and toxic dilatation of the colon. Investigations include malabsorption and infection screens, double-contrast barium enema, colonoscopy and biopsies.

Management of both conditions involves a high-energy, low-fibre diet with vitamin supplements and drugs (eg mesalazine or sulfasalazine) associated with immunosuppressive agents, such as steroids. Surgery is indicated in Crohn's disease only if there are complications such as bowel obstruction or perforation. However, in ulcerative colitis, surgery may be required for failure to respond to conservative treatment, toxic dilatation, severe gastrointestinal bleeding or perforation, and ultimately as prophylaxis against its associated increased risk of malignancy.

4.26 B, D

Precocious puberty is defined as the onset of sexual maturation before 8 years in a girl and 9 years in a boy. It is at least four times more common in girls and usually no cause is found. However, in boys it is essential to investigate because, in 80–90% of cases, a cause is found (eg intracranial tumour). The most important sequela is decreased final height, because the initial associated growth spurt is short-lived and the advanced bone age results in early epiphyseal fusion.

Important investigations include skull radiograph, bone age, CT of the head, urinary 17-ketosteroids, pelvic ultrasonography and TFTs. Management involves referral to a specialist for treatment aiming to achieve constant high levels of synthetic gonadotrophin-releasing hormone (GnRH) analogues in the circulation. This 'non-pulsatile' regimen paradoxically suppresses the secretion of pituitary gonadotrophins, which reverses gonadal and slows skeletal maturation. Treatment should be continued until the average age of puberty (ie 11 years) and parents should be reassured that the child will develop normally.

Features of McCune–Albright syndrome include polyosteotic fibrous dysplasia of bone, irregular areas of skin pigmentation, and facial asymmetry with or without precocious puberty. Coeliac disease is associated with delayed puberty.

4.27 B

Bow legs (genu varum) are normal in infants and usually correct by 3 years of age. Knock-knees (genu valgum) are normal up to about 5 years. Predisposing conditions include osteogenesis imperfecta, rickets, Blount's disease (infantile tibia vara) and chondrodysplasia. Genu varum also results from medial tibial torsion; this usually spontaneously corrects within 5 years and no treatment is required. However, forward bowing is pathological (eg rickets) and active management is essential. Osgood–Schlatter disease occurs with inflammation of the tibial tuberosity at the insertion of the patellar tendon and results in painful knees. Neither bow legs nor knock-knees are a feature, although the latter is a common sequela of poliomyelitis.

answers

4.28 B, D, E

A normal 18-month-old infant can kick a ball forward; this develops between 15 months and 2 years. He or she can walk backwards from about 1 year and climb upstairs holding on, but uses two feet per step. They cannot balance on one foot because this develops later at around 22 months to 3 years. 'Bottom shufflers' may be delayed walkers, although most infants walk well by 14 months.

4.29 B

Neither HIV nor AIDS is a notifiable disease. The risk of vertical transmission in Europe is between 13% and 25% and has been shown to decrease with antiviral drugs in pregnancy and caesarean section, although this figure is much higher in Africa. Testing neonates for the presence of HIV antibodies is not helpful in excluding a congenital infection because of the transmission of maternal antibodies. However, p24 antigen and polymerase chain reaction are of use. Although the risk of transmission via breast milk is small, where safe alternatives are available breast-feeding should be avoided. However, in developing countries the risks of breast-feeding far outweigh the benefits of the alternatives and should therefore be encouraged. Note that HIV is a positive indication for pneumococcal immunisation.

4.30 B, E

Many 3-year-olds are 'dry' both day and night. They can feed, wash and dress themselves without supervision, including donning shoes, but are unable to manage complex buckles or laces. They will interact with other children in both imaginary and non-imaginary play.

4.31 A, B, C, E

Most 3-year-old children can recognise three colours, know their full name and will use over 200 words in conversation. However, they can only define about six words from around 3–4 years, but will comprehend the meaning of various sensations, such as cold/tired/hungry.

answers

4.32 C, D, E

Ten per cent of affected children present with irreducible inguinal hernias, with an increased incidence in the first 3 months. Prompt elective surgery is essential before 1 year of age to prevent obstruction and strangulation.

4.33 C, E

Mesenteric adenitis often follows an URTI and is associated with lymphadenopathy elsewhere, especially in the cervical and axillary nodes. It presents with poorly localised, intermittent abdominal pain with no signs of peritonitis and often a high pyrexia (38°C) and lymphocytosis. It may be recurrent. It is frequently caused by an adenovirus and treatment with simple analgesia is sufficient.

4.34 A, C, E

Edwards syndrome (trisomy 18) is associated with hypertonicity, low-set malformed ears, receding chin, protruding eyes, cleft lip/palate, rocker bottom feet and umbilical/inguinal herniae. Expected survival is approximately 10 months.

Laurence–Moon–Biedl syndrome is an autosomal recessive condition that mainly affects boys. It presents with night blindness, progressing to visual loss. Other features include obesity, polydactyly, small genitals, paraparesis, decreased IQ, retinitis pigmentosa, squint and cataract.

Noonan syndrome is an autosomal dominant condition with a 1 in 5000 prevalence. Any system may be affected, but common associations include heart defects (eg hypertrophic cardiomyopathy/septal defects), ptosis, downward slanting eyes, low-set ears and a webbed neck. There may be a coagulopathy and slightly reduced height and IQ.

Pierre Robin syndrome presents with neonatal difficulty with feeding and breathing secondary to micrognathia (short chin) ± cleft palate.

Turner's syndrome (XO) has a prevalence of 1 in 2500 girls and is associated with short stature, a wide carrying angle (cubitus valgus), webbed neck, coarctation of the aorta, and rudimentary or absent gonads.

4.35 B, C, D, E

Language delay has an increased occurrence among boys and girls from large families – with first-born and only children being the least likely to be affected. Other associated features include developmental delay, deafness, autism and abnormalities of the speech apparatus, ie neurological (eg cerebral palsy) and physical (eg cleft palate – secondary to dysarthria and recurrent otitis media). Severe language delay has as an incidence of 1 in 1000.

Speech and language therapists can accurately assess children aged between 1 and 5 years using Reynell's Developmental Language Scale, to see whether the delay is the result of comprehension, expression or both. Management depends on the cause and may involve a multidisciplinary approach, including audiology, orthodontic referral, plastic surgery or simply speech and language therapy alone.

answers

Answers to Extending Matching Questions

4.36 Essential nutrients

1   I – Vitamin E

Ataxia and weakness are signs of vitamin E deficiency. Vitamin E is routinely supplemented in children with cystic fibrosis. This is because vitamin E is fat soluble (along with vitamins A, D and K) and may be malabsorbed as a result of exocrine pancreatic deficiency.

2   F – Vitamin B_{12}

Folic acid deficiency is unlikely in a vegan diet because green vegetables and legumes are good sources. Vitamin B_{12} is, however, mainly obtained from dairy products and meat products, and deficiency results in megaloblastic anaemia. Treatment with vitamin B_{12} supplements stimulates a good bone marrow response.

3   H – Vitamin D

Vitamin D deficiency leads to reduced calcium uptake from the gut. Calcium is reabsorbed (stimulated by parathyroid hormone or PTH) from the bone to maintain serum levels. Alkaline phosphatase (ALP) levels are characteristically increased, reflecting osteoclastic activity. These biochemical changes progress to clinical rickets with prominent wrists (caused by the 'cupped, splayed, frayed' appearance of the radial and ulnar metaphyses, and those of the other long bones). A 'rachitic rosary' may be present as a result of swelling of the costochondral junctions. Treatment is with vitamin D supplementation.

4.37 Respiratory conditions

1   D – Foreign body inhalation

In a toddler who presents with sudden and/or recent difficulty in breathing, foreign body aspiration must always be considered, especially if initially associated with a choking episode. Toddlers are inquisitive and will put most small objects in their mouths. Any asymmetry in chest signs such as expansion or wheeze should increase the index of suspicion.

2   G – Pertussis

An immunisation history must always be requested in addition to reviewing the personal child health record or 'red book'. Classic features of whooping cough include a cough that occurs in paroxysms, associated with vomiting, subconjunctival haemorrhages from repeated coughing and a marked lymphocytosis. Treatment is supportive but erythromycin can be given to limit infectivity to other children. The cough can last up to 3 months (the 100-day cough).

3   B – Atopic asthma

A previous history of an atopic condition or a family history of atopy increases the risk of asthma (and other atopic conditions). A nocturnal cough is a recognised presentation of asthma in pre-school children. A trial of an inhaled bronchodilator via a spacer is worthwhile.

answers

4.38 Gastrointestinal disorders

1   D – Crohn's disease

The history and objective weight loss suggest significant pathology. The time course is a little lengthy to be infective, although not impossible. The inflammatory markers are raised, indicating an ongoing inflammatory process. The perianal skin tags should strongly raise the suspicion of Crohn's disease. This disease is increasing in childhood, with current incidence being between 10 and 25 per 100,000. It is an inflammatory process involving the whole bowel (mouth to anus). Clinically, patients present with abdominal pain, weight loss/reduced growth and diarrhoea. On examination there may be mouth ulceration and perianal lesions. Extra-gastrointestinal features may be present, including arthralgia, anaemia and uveitis. Investigations include endoscopy and possibly radiological contrast studies. Treatment should be shared among a tertiary level, multidisciplinary, paediatric gastroenterological team and secondary and primary care.

2   H – Toddler's diarrhoea

This is a classic history for toddler's diarrhoea. The child is well and thriving but the parents can understandably be anxious. The cause is thought to be the result of a fast enteric transit time and a brisk gastrocolic reflex. Reassurance is vital, but simple measures such as reducing fruit juice intake may help.

3   J – Viral gastroenteritis

This is an acute history so an infective process is likely; the fact that her sibling had a similar illness again makes an infective cause much more likely. A viral cause is more common in this age group (eg rotavirus). Viral gastroenteritis is a self-limiting condition but there is a risk of dehydration if oral intake is insufficient. Medications such as loperamide or codeine to 'reduce' the diarrhoea have no place in management, and may lengthen the duration of the illness. Secondary lactose intolerance is uncommon and, before changing the milk to a lactose-free formula, stool-reducing sugars should be checked.

4.39 Endocrine disorders

1   I – Small genetic height potential

This child may not have a big genetic height potential (ie her overall potential height determined by her genes if both her parents are not tall). It is unlikely that she will be tall.

2   C – Constitutional delay in growth and puberty

There are no clinical signs of puberty yet in this boy, except that his testicular volume is 8 mL. The pubertal growth spurt normally starts once the testicular volume reaches 10 mL. The delayed bone age means that there is still growth potential in the bones, so that, if the bone age is delayed by 2 years, once puberty starts he will have an 'extra' 2 years of growth compared with his peers. Constitutional delay of growth and puberty can be managed with reassurance; however, peer pressure and bullying at school may lead some families to want intervention. In these cases a short course of testosterone may 'kick start' the growth.

3   F – Hypothyroidism

The features of constipation, weight gain and academic faltering are consistent with hypothyroidism. Acquired hypothyroidism is the result of two main causes: autoimmune (Hashimoto's) thyroiditis and post-total body irradiation (TBI). Worldwide the most common cause is iodine deficiency. As part of the preparation for bone marrow transplantation requires TBI, this is the most likely cause. Treatment is with thyroxine replacement.

4.40 Neurodevelopmental and psychological problems

1   D – Autism

Autism is an increasing problem. It was first described by Kanner in 1943, and is a triad of communication difficulties, socialisation problems and attention problems. This 3-year-old shows poor language skills and poor eye contact (socialisation problem). The features of autism are mostly present before the age of 2 years, but the diagnosis may not necessarily be made at that time. The language difficulties can be profound and up to 30% of autistic children may never develop language. Treatment modalities include speech and language therapy, behavioural therapy to improve socialisation and attention.

2   G – Psychosocial deprivation

In a child who was previously thriving but is now growth faltering, and who has some developmental delay, the diagnosis of psychosocial deprivation must always be considered. This is a diagnosis of exclusion, once organic causes have been ruled out. In this case there are other warning signs of this diagnosis – she has missed some immunisations, she will play games (so probably has no socialisation difficulties) and her dentition is poor, a possible sign of neglect.

3   H – Post-traumatic stress disorder

Post-traumatic stress disorder (PTSD), although still uncommon, is an increasing diagnosis in paediatric psychiatry. The trauma of sexual assault has led to the behavioural problems in this girl. PTSD can be caused by sexual assault, physical assault or indeed any experience of very traumatic situations (eg refugees from a conflict zone). It can present in a myriad of ways: concentration difficulties, mood instability, aggression, flashbacks, sleep disturbance, anxiety, depression and parasuicide. Cognitive–behavioural therapy and counselling may help disclosure of the trigger, and provide effective results.

answers

4.41 Special investigations

1   D – Echocardiogram

The single most important late complication of Kawasaki's disease is development of coronary artery aneurysms. An echocardiogram, in skilled hands, is an easy, simple and effective way of detecting aneurysms. An angiogram is sometimes performed in tertiary paediatric cardiac centres, to further demonstrate aneurysms seen on the echocardiogram.

2   C– CT

Any seizure after a head injury is an indication for further imaging. A skull radiograph may reveal a skull fracture, but given the fact that there has been a seizure brain imaging is required. CT of the brain is quick to do and readily available and is the investigation of choice in the NICE guidelines for the management of a head injury.

3   G – MRI

The concern in this child is that there may be an underlying osteomyelitis. A plain film may reveal some periosteal reaction, but only if the infection has been present for over 1 week. A bone scan was previously the investigation of choice, with the infection showing as a hot spot at the site of the infection. However, MRI is now the imaging modality of choice – it will show periosteal and intramedullary oedema as well as the anatomical detail of soft tissue changes and any joint involvement. It is recognised that MRI may be technically difficult in some age groups and not available in some centres, and a bone scan may be performed in these situations.

answers

4.42 Rashes

1   A – Milia

Milia affect the nose, zygomatic skin and forehead. They are as described – pinpoint white spots that are present from birth. It is a benign condition.

2   D – Staphylococcal septic spots

The most common rash in the neonatal period is erythema toxicum; however, it is important not to forget that this classically appears on the face and trunk. Yellow pustules in the groin, neck and axillary flexures are more likely to be staphylococcal in origin. The umbilical stump should be inspected if staphylococcal lesions are present because this may also be infected and have a red 'flare' around it. The treatment for this is intravenous flucloxacillin.

3   F – Infantile acne

This condition is normally described in baby boys aged 3–6 months. Classically affecting the cheeks, forehead and chin, it is an eruption of comedones (blackheads and whiteheads) and also pustular eruptions. It is sometimes said to be caused by hormonal changes. It can be distinguished from neonatal acne by the history (neonatal acne occurs before 3 months) and the fact that neonatal acne is only a pustular rash. Treatment of infantile acne is with benzoyl peroxide or occasionally oral antibiotics. This condition can lead to permanent scarring, so it should not be underestimated.

4.43 Healthcare roles

1   H – Speech and language therapist

Children on the autistic spectrum have a disorder of communication, socialisation and behaviour. The approach to a child with autism has to be multidisciplinary, and the diagnosis is ideally made in a combined assessment of paediatrician, psychologist and speech and language therapist. In the child in question, there is input into his care from a psychologist and an educational psychologist, but a speech and language therapist is not listed. Speech and language therapy is vital to maximise communication potential (not just speech).

2   G – Orthotist

This child is having contractures as a result of her cerebral palsy. Physiotherapy is key to the prevention of contractures and alleviation. However, splinting is an important part of the care of this condition. Splints allow passive stretching of the splinted joint and may allow better function. As an example, a child with tight Achilles' tendons may not be able to walk because the angle of the toes causes tripping; if the foot is splinted then the Achilles' tendons will be stretched and the angle improved, allowing walking without tripping.

3   E – Occupational therapist

Children with juvenile idiopathic arthritis (JIA) often need help with day-to-day activities, especially at school. Occupational therapists can advise the school (in conjunction with a physiotherapist) on what is necessary to provide easier access for the child and (in conjunction with the educational psychologist) can give input on strategies to make learning easier – using 'fat' pens that are easier to grip and a laptop with voice recognition software are two examples.

answers

Best of Five Answers

4.44 D

It is fundamental step to assess what he is actually doing in comparison to the therapeutic plan that has been made, ie if he is taking preventive medication very infrequently, if at all. Inadequate adherence to an effective management plan is a common problem in many children, especially during adolescence.

4.45 C

Urticaria and mild angio-oedema may be triggered by various allergens such as food allergens, or physical factors such as pressure, cold, etc. A food and symptom diary may well identify a pattern of a food or food ingredient that is closely associated in time to the development of these symptoms, and is a reasonable initial action with few adverse effects. Regular use of a sedating antihistamine for such an infrequent and mild symptom is not likely to be an acceptable strategy. Topical steroids are of no value in treating this condition. Urticaria is not a feature of hereditary angio-oedema. A milk, egg or wheat allergy is very unlikely to produce infrequent symptoms such as these at this age, and such a diet is not an easy strategy.

4.46 D

The episodes consist of sudden brief loss of posture and awareness, with rapid recovery, and appear to be precipitated when active. They do not typify generalised epilepsy. There is no associated precipitant such as a painful knock or temper tantrum. The twitching noted may occur with syncopal attacks whatever the cause. However, the family history is significant and points to a possible inherited abnormality. A resting ECG, possibly with continuous 24-hour monitoring, is needed to identify an arrhythmia, which is the diagnosis. An exercise ECG may also be helpful in the long QT syndrome, the proven diagnosis.

4.47 B

This girl is most likely to be suffering from inflammatory bowel disease, probably ulcerative colitis. The most valuable investigation that will give an assessment of severity and extent of the disease is a colonoscopy. Barium studies and abdominal radiographs do not give sufficient information. Radio-isotope scans will help in identifying an abnormality such as Meckel's diverticulum and angiography is rarely indicated, unless a vascular lesion is suspected of leading to an intestinal bleed.

4.48 D

This baby had a probable viral respiratory illness and the presence of healing rib fractures was an unexpected finding on the chest radiograph. The presence of well-formed callus dates the occurrence of the fractures to 1–2 weeks before the radiograph. Antenatal accidents as causes of fractures are extremely rare and can be discounted if the mother had no major injuries. In addition, considering the age of the baby, the callus should have completely resolved. Severe pertussis may rarely be the cause of a rib fracture, but this is not compatible with the presentation. Social Services need to be involved and are likely to organise a strategy meeting before discharge.

4.49 E

This child's initial developmental progress was normal but he is now having a progressive neurological problem with difficulty in gait. Thus, by definition, this is not cerebral palsy. Guillain–Barré syndrome is characterised by the development of ascending muscle weakness after a febrile illness. Myasthenia gravis is characterised by progressive muscular fatigue. Becker's muscular dystrophy has a later onset than the Duchenne type, in which a Gower's manoeuvre is a common finding in association with calf hypertrophy.

4.50 D

This child has had two acute lung infections affecting the same area of the lung in a period of 9 months. The history suggests that she recovered fully after the first attack and had been well in the intervening period. However, the original radiograph was not available, although a copy of the report was seen. The history does not suggest a chronic respiratory problem and the most logical step is to review her response to antibiotics both clinically and radiologically before further investigations are instigated. In the presence of recurrent clinical and/or radiological abnormality, elimination of a foreign body, chronic infection, eg TB, pulmonary sequestration and immune deficiency may need to be considered.

4.51 B

The failure to thrive, recurrent respiratory infections, oral ulcers, recurrent ear discharge and intermittent diarrhoea are most likely to be associated with an immune deficiency. This diagnosis is supported by low IgA level and a relatively low IgG level and low lymphocyte count. The coeliac screen is negative, but not excluded because of the low IgA, although it is unlikely with a history of mouth ulcers and the finding of a normal serum ferritin. Children with toddler's diarrhoea thrive satisfactorily and lactose intolerance is associated with explosive diarrhoea.

4.52 D

Thyroid function tests should be performed at birth (as part of the Guthrie card), at 12 months and again at 3 years of age. Children with Down's syndrome should have their height and weight plotted on specific Down's syndrome growth charts. Urine tests are not part of routine screening unless there is a clinical indication. Dental screening should start at 18 months. Additional screening includes eye checks for visual behaviour and squints at 6 weeks, 6 months and 1 year, followed by an orthoptic review at 2 and 4 years. Full audiological review is performed at 6, 12 and 18 months, as well as at 4 years.

answers

4.53 E

This child has presented with a likely spontaneous haemarthrosis. The treatment of choice is factor VIII infusion. Recurrent haemarthroses can lead to erosion and the eventual need for replacement of the joint. Platelet transfusion and vitamin K have little role in the treatment of haemophilia A. Desmopressin (DDAVP) is used in the milder forms of the disease often for home treatment administered by a nasal spray. DDAVP stimulates endogenous factor VIII release; however, an individual's response to DDAVP should be assessed before routine use.

4.54 D

Jaundice at less than 24 h of age is pathological. Dehydration is highly unlikely at this age, and would have responded to intravenous fluids. ABO incompatibility is not a consideration in a mother who is group AB because she will have no anti-A or anti-B antibodies. Rhesus haemolytic disease occurs in only rhesus-negative mothers. Gilbert's disease presents later in life. G6PDH deficiency is the most likely explanation, especially given the fact that it happened to an older male sibling.

4.55 A

Positional plagiocephaly is increasingly seen. This is probably a result of the 'back to sleep' campaign. The condition is completely benign; however, understandably, it causes parents a degree of anxiety. Placing toys on the other side of the cot works well early on, but less well at this age. Most neurosurgical units offer no intervention but do offer parent information sheets. There is no evidence that moulding helmets affect the course of this spontaneously resolving condition. Tempting as it might be to place the child on his front to sleep, this would increase the risk of SIDS and be against all advice.

4.56 E

Abdominal pain is a presenting feature in 20% of children with diabetic ketoacidosis. There are various possible diagnoses for this child; however, few are likely to lead to 10% dehydration. Of the investigations listed, only a blood glucose will lead to a diagnosis. An arterial blood gas will show the degree and type of acidosis but not the underlying cause. A CRP and FBC may well be abnormal, but again will not help with the underlying cause.

4.57 E

Although malathion and permethrin are commonly used treatments for head lice, neither is recommended for children aged under 2. Carbaryl is a strong insecticide that is reserved only for resistant cases. Wet combing is effective and 'bug-busting kits' are available on the NHS; it is also less drastic than shaving heads.

It is important also to treat all other affected family members.

4.58 E

The new vaccine is equally efficacious as the old vaccine and, as part of the five-in-one vaccine, more convenient. There was variability in the virulence and excretion of the live attenuated virus, which always needed to be considered if there was an immunocompromised individual in close contact. The main reason for the change in schedule was that there were indeed more cases of vaccine polio than wild polio.

4.59 D

GHB causes relaxation and, in larger doses, coma. It is found in a liquid preparation. The effects of overdose are as described. Cannabis overdose is uncommon and unlikely to cause such a reduced conscious level. Amyl nitrate causes an intense vasodilatation and few problems are reported in overdose, although arrhythmias are recorded. Cocaine is a stimulant that causes sympathetic stimulation in overdose; an important side effect of cocaine is coronary artery spasm, which is a recognised cause of myocardial infarction in young children. Ecstasy causes an increase in serotonin levels. In overdose sympathetic overdrive occurs and a malignant hyperthermia occurs – this is the common cause of death. (An excellent review of recreational drugs can be found in *Archives of Disease in Childhood 2006;91*:3.)

4.60 B

A spiking fever and conjunctivitis would be expected in periorbital cellulitis. A headache is a non-specific sign that might occur, but it could cause concern if it persisted. Loss of pupillary reflex is a sign that an orbital cellulitis or preseptal abscess is developing, both of which require urgent assessment by an ophthalmologist.

4.61 A

Prebiotics are fructo- and malto-oligosaccharides that act as 'food' for natural gut flora. This preferential growth of normal flora is considered to have an immunomodulating effect. Although all the other points are proposed benefits for prebiotics, there is scanty evidence for this at present. There is some evidence in the form of a randomised controlled trial that showed a reduction in atopic dermatitis.

4.62 D

The clinical signs exhibited by this child are consistent with heart failure. The investigation most likely to inform the diagnosis is an echocardiogram. An important consideration in any child who has received treatment for any neoplasm is the possibility of a relapse, which would not be an unreasonable diagnosis (because severe anaemia can cause heart failure); however, the FBC is normal and that makes it very unlikely. A chest radiograph would probably show cardiomegaly, but little else of use. An echocardiogram would show poor left ventricular function which is a result of doxorubicin-induced cardiomyopathy – an important treatment side effect.

4.63 E

Antidepressant medication for children should be started only by a child and adolescent psychiatrist as part of a multidisciplinary strategy. Medication should be started only after four to six sessions of psychological therapy have not helped. Tricyclic antidepressants such as amitriptyline should not be used in childhood depression; there are better treatments available that are far safer in overdose. Diazepam has a limited role in inpatient treatment. Paroxetine, a selective serotonin reuptake inhibitor (SSRI), should not be used in the treatment of children aged under 18; there is increased risk of self-harm and suicidal behaviour. Fluoxetine is recommended as the first-line treatment and sertraline as a second-line treatment.

4.64 D

A bacterial abscess on the scalp is uncommon in children, unless immunocompromised. In the unlikely event that a bacterial abscess does develop, the lesion is very painful and the child is often systemically unwell.

The preceding rash is tinea capitis. The lesion described in this child is a kerion, which is an inflammatory mass caused by a fungal scalp infection. The lesion is filled with pus and often mistaken for a bacterial abscess, leading to incision and drainage; this will have no impact on the underlying process and may result in subsequent patches of hair loss. Treatment is with systemic antifungals and antibiotics. Dermatology opinions should be obtained early in the management.

answers

4.65 C

The cause of the gross haematuria associated with renal colic may be a nephroblastoma (Wilms' tumour) which sometimes may not be palpable. The quickest and most relevant examination is an ultrasound examination of the kidneys, lower ureters and bladder. If this indicates any renal mass abnormality then CT is done. Renal stones are rare in this age group but may well be detectable on ultrasound examination. Metabolic analysis will be required if the diagnosis of renal calculi is positive. MAG-3 scan is useful if there is any evidence of ureteric obstruction.

4.66 D

The most relevant investigation is MRI. The first seizure in a child with significant headache needs urgent evaluation, preferably by MRI, because some space-occupying lesions could be missed on CT. The absence of vomiting, early morning headaches, neurological changes and normal optic discs does not exclude an early diagnosis of a cerebral tumour. The EEG may indicate a focal lesion, but if normal does not exclude a significant brain lesion. The diagnosis of migraine in the above circumstances should be by elimination of the above and pizotifen is not an investigation.

4.67 C

All the given causes could cause bruising, the first four being potential causes of thrombocytopenia. However, the clinical, haematological, bone marrow and immunological findings are most compatible with ITP. Although she had a 'viral' illness it was very unlikely to have been glandular fever. The marrow and haematology did not have any features of ALL or drug-induced bone marrow suppression. The presence of an anti-platelet antibody (PaIgG) is usually not important in diagnosing ITP.

4.68 D

This girl has a tendency to leak urine involuntarily in spite of regular bladder emptying and use of the toilet, so it is not primary enuresis. The mild vulvitis is the result of dribbling rather than the cause of it. Although there is a history of temper tantrums, there is no evidence of ongoing behaviour difficulties or major 'accidental wetting'. The observation of urine trickling continuously at the introitus could be the result only of an ectopic ureter of a duplex system. VUR is associated with recurrent UTIs, and loss of bladder control is associated with urgency and dysuria.

THE DCH CLINICAL EXAMINATION

The new Diploma of Child Health clinical examination was introduced in March 2006. The standard expected is that of a newly qualified general practitioner. There are six different types of stations, two of which are repeated, giving a total of eight stations. All stations are observed by an examiner. It is essential to read the detailed information about the DCH examination on the Royal College of Paediatrics' website (www.rcpch.ac.uk) in the 'Exams' section. This gives information about the stations, and how the examination is run and assessed. An approach to vision and hearing testing is given. In addition, read the information for examiners because this will give you a valuable insight into what is expected – it is not a secret!

The six different stations are:

1   Focused history taking and care planning (13 min)

2   Communication skills (two stations of 5 min each)

3   Structured oral (13 min)

4   Short clinical cases (two stations of 5 min each)

5   Clinical neurodisability (13 min)

6   Child development (13 min).

GENERAL TIPS ON COMMUNICATION AND EXAMINING CHILDREN

The examiners rightly put great importance on having a child-friendly approach. Always be polite, professional and empathic.

You should talk to and examine the child in a way that puts him or her at ease, but be confident. Your approach should be appropriate for their age and development:

- Introduce yourself to the child and parent and explain what you are doing.

- Ask the child's name and age and use his or her name during the case.

- Avoid using medical jargon, abbreviations, or worrying or pejorative words.

- Careful observation is often the most important part of the examination in a young child. Use it to get as much information as you can before proceeding.

- Always ask about pain and examine a child gently. Never cause any pain or be rough.

- Position and expose the child appropriately but don't embarrass him or her. A young child (younger than 3 years) is best examined on the parent's knee. An older child should be examined on a couch.

- Clean your hands and stethoscope between patients.

- Present your findings in a structured way.

The approach to the examination of a child varies with the child's age and development. An older child should be examined in a structured and systematic way following the standard adult approach. In a young child (pre-school) the examination will need to be opportunistic and flexible according to how the child behaves, eg percussion of the chest is often not useful in an infant and may upset him or her. Use age-appropriate toys for play and distraction and get down to the child's level. You will develop these skills only by practising examining children of different ages. Most candidates find it helpful to talk as they go along because silence is often awkward. State the obvious things that you see, eg scars or tubes, but do not commit yourself to uncertain signs until you have had time to put all the information together.

FOCUSED HISTORY TAKING AND CARE PLANNING STATION

In this station you have 8 min to take a focused history from a child and parent while being observed, followed by questions on the case for 5 min. You may be given other information such as a growth chart. The child will usually have a chronic disease. This is not a test of whether you can take a 'full' history, but whether you can focus on the current problems and key issues for the child and family. Imagine that you are in an outpatient consultation with the family for the first time:

- Introduce yourself and establish rapport with the child and parent.

- The history taking should be structured.

- Start with open questions, then focus with closed questions.

- Ensure that you understand the key psychological, social and educational issues.

- Use a quick checklist of headings so that you don't miss anything important, eg past medical history, medication, immunisations and development.

- Determine which members of the multidisciplinary team the child sees.

- What are the family's main worries and concerns?

- Summarise the problems to the parent to ensure that you have obtained all the key information.

- Decide what are the management priorities, including further investigations and referrals.

- Practise taking focused histories for the common chronic illnesses in the allocated time.

EXAMPLES

Case 1: asthma

Problem: a 10-year-boy with poorly controlled asthma.

- Determine current asthma symptoms, persistence and severity
- Frequency and nature of exacerbations, number of hospital attendances, courses of oral steroids
- Effect on exercise, sleep and schooling
- Triggers, eg smoking, pets
- Current treatment, inhalers and devices
- Psychosocial factors impacting on illness
- Side effects of steroids, eg poor growth
- Management issues
- How was asthma diagnosed? Could it be something else?
- Peak flow monitoring
- Inhaler technique and compliance
- Environmental measures, eg house-dust mite avoidance
- Add-on therapies, eg long-acting β agonists.

Case 2: cerebral palsy

Problem: a 5-year-old girl (ex-premature) with spastic diplegia.

- Perinatal and developmental history important
- Determine what the child can do functionally
- Determine associated problems, eg seizures, visual problems, constipation
- Are there associated learning and behavioural problems?
- Determine mobility, eg joint contractures, special aids and splints
- Multidisciplinary team input. Who and how often, eg physiotherapist, social worker, educational psychologist?
- Respite care and support
- Education.

Common cases are diabetes, ex-premature infant with chronic lung disease, cystic fibrosis, inflammatory bowel disease, nephrotic syndrome, congenital heart disease and muscular dystrophy.

the clinical examination

COMMUNICATION SKILLS STATION

- You are given a scenario to communicate with a parent, older child or health professional.

- You will be given information about your role and the clinical background.

- Introduce yourself and explain your role.

- Allow the parent or child time to speak.

- Explore their concerns and expectations.

- Ensure that the information you give is appropriate and accurate.

- Be aware of the emotional context of the situation and show empathy, eg anxious parent.

- Summarise and check understanding of the important issues.

Possible scenarios

Information giving
- Explain the diagnosis of 'febrile convulsion' to a mother whose child has just had a fit.

- Explain the principles of management of diabetes to a newly diagnosed adolescent.

Consent
- Obtain consent from a parent to perform a lumbar puncture on a child with meningitis.

Critical incident
- Talk to a parent whose child received the wrong dose of an antibiotic in error.

Education
- Explain to a parent how to give buccal midazolam for seizures.

Explanation of medical devices

●   Explain to a school nurse how to use an EpiPen for anaphylaxis.

Difficult or 'bad news' scenarios

●   You see a child with bruising, which you suspect may be non-accidental. What do you say to the parent?

●   You see an infant who you diagnose clinically as having Down's syndrome. Discuss your findings with the parents.

the clinical examination

STRUCTURED ORAL STATION

You will be tested on two common child health problems or topics. You may be asked about acute or chronic problems and community child health. Examples:

- Assessment of dehydration
- Management of acute seizures
- Management of the child with a purpuric rash
- Assessment of short stature or precocious puberty
- Management of constipation, diabetes or nocturnal enuresis
- Management and complications of childhood obesity
- Immunisation topics, eg current schedule, special groups
- Child protection, eg recognition, referral procedures
- Diagnosis of autism.

SHORT CLINICAL CASES STATION

You will be tested on two system examinations, eg cardiovascular, respiratory, abdomen, endocrine system, growth, skin and joints.

In each case general observation of the child's activity, appearance (any dysmorphism), nutrition and growth is important. Look for any medicines or equipment that may give clues to the diagnosis. In general you should follow the classic schema below, starting with general observation, then proceeding to the hands and head. The approach in younger children will need to be more flexible as previously stated.

- Inspection/Observation

- Palpation

- Percussion

- Auscultation.

Examination of the cardiovascular system

Observation

- Is the child dysmorphic, eg Down's syndrome, Turner's syndrome?

- Know the cardiac defects that occur in common syndromes, eg AVSD (Atrio-ventricular septal defect)/ventricular septal defect (VSD) in Down's syndrome

- Tachypnoea or respiratory distress.

Hands

- Look for clubbing

- Feel both brachial pulses

- Determine the rate, rhythm and character of the pulse

- State that you would measure the blood pressure and know how to.

the clinical examination

Face

- Assess the lips and tongue for central cyanosis
- Anaemia or polycythaemia.

Chest

- Look for scars, eg axillary or central sternotomy.

Palpation

- Locate the apex beat and assess if normally positioned
- Make sure that you can feel the apex on the left, otherwise there may be dextrocardia
- Feel for parasternal heave and thrills.

Auscultation

- Listen in the four cardiac areas and at the back
- Listen to the second heart sound. Is it loud or abnormally split? (Normally widens with inspiration)
- Are there additional sounds, eg clicks or murmurs?
- For a murmur determine:

    – timing, eg systolic (ejection or pansystolic), diastolic or continuous

    – character

    – grade and where it is loudest (grade 4 and above associated with thrill is always pathological)

    – radiation

    – change with position or respiration

- Note that outflow tract murmurs (aortic or pulmonary) are loudest above the nipple line.

Additional

- Feel the femoral pulses
- Palpate for a liver in a young child.

Common cases

- VSD, pulmonary stenosis, aortic stenosis, patent ductus arteriosus, atrial septal defect, dextrocardia
- Child with congenital heart disease that has been corrected, eg transposition or Fallot's tetralogy
- Know how to distinguish an innocent from a pathological murmur.

Examination of the respiratory system

Observation

- Signs of respiratory distress and count the respiratory rate
- Look for inhalers, pancreatic enzymes, sputum
- Listen for cough, stridor or wheeze.

Hands

- Clubbing (implies bronchiectasis or cystic fibrosis)
- Pulse rate.

Head

- Central cyanosis, anaemia
- Feel for cervical lymph nodes.

Chest

- Look for hyperinflation (increased anterior–posterior diameter), a sign of asthma or chronic lung disease
- Look for asymmetry
- Harrison's sulci
- Scars.

the clinical examination

Palpation

- Assess for mediastinal shift by gently palpating for tracheal deviation suprasternally and locate the apex beat

- Assess chest expansion.

Percussion

- Anterior, axilla and posterior

- Percussion note

- Less useful in infants and toddlers.

Auscultation

- Anterior, axilla and posterior

- Listen to the breath sounds and for additional sounds (wheezes and crackles). Breath sounds can be normal (vesicular), absent, reduced or bronchial. Are they symmetrical?

- Vocal resonance if you suspect consolidation

- Examine the front first then the back in a structured way (four places at the front, both axillae and six places at the back)

- Describe your findings according to upper, middle and lower zones.

Additional things

- Say that you wish to examine the ears, nose and throat

- Measure the peak flow

- Palpate and percuss the liver.

Common cases

- Chronic asthma, cystic fibrosis, bronchiectasis, ex-premature infant with chronic lung disease, child with previous tracheostomy.

Examination of the abdomen

Observation

- Signs of chronic liver disease, eg spider naevi
- Comment on nasogastric tubes and gastrostomies.

Hands

- Clubbing
- Palmar erythema.

Face

- Sclera for jaundice
- Mouth for ulcers
- Conjunctiva for anaemia.

Abdomen

- Adequate exposure while maintaining dignity of the child
- Assess for abdominal distension
- Scars: look at the back.

Palpation

- Ask the child if he or she has any abdominal pain
- Gentle palpation of the four quadrants followed by deeper palpation
- Look at the child's face the whole time to ensure that you are not causing pain (you do not need to look at your hand!)
- Examine for an enlarged liver and a spleen starting in the right iliac fossa
- Measure the size of any enlarged organ or mass
- To examine for a mildly enlarged spleen lie the child on his or her right side
- Examine for palpable kidneys by bimanual ballottement

- If there is distension, test for ascites by shifting dullness and a fluid thrill.

Percussion
- Percuss the four quadrants and the upper and lower borders of an enlarged organ.

Ausculation
- Listen for bowel sounds and bruits.

In addition:
- Say that you would inspect the genitalia, perianal area and hernial orifices
- Measure the blood pressure (renal disease)
- Obtain urine for dipstick.

Common cases
- Know the causes of hepatomegaly and splenomegaly
- Splenomegaly may be the result of haematological causes (hereditary spherocytosis, sickle cell disease), storage diseases, portal hypertension, malignancy and infections
- Polycystic kidney or pelvic kidney (transplant), nephrotic syndrome
- Biliary atresia post-Kasai procedure and liver transplantation.

Examination of the joints

Observation
- Look for joint swelling, erythema, deformity, wasting and scars
- Number and distribution of joints involved if arthritis.

Palpation
- Feel for warmth, tenderness, swelling (eg patellar tap) and crepitus

- Swelling may be a joint effusion, synovial thickening, soft tissue or bony.

Move
- Ask if there is pain before moving
- Assess the range of movement of the joint; it may be limited by pain, contracture or spasticity; compare both sides
- First active movements by the child, then passive movements assessed by you
- Assess function
- Measure limb length
- Examine the spine for scoliosis.

Examination of the skin
- Expose appropriately; describe what you see
- Describe the shape of the skin lesions; palpate the lesions.
- Types of lesion: macular, papular, vesicular, haemangioma
- Colour of the lesion: hypo- or hyperpigmentation, purpura, erythema
- Distribution of lesions, eg localised or generalised, symmetrical, flexural
- Signs of itching and excoriation
- Look at the mouth, teeth, nails, eg pitting, and hair, eg alopecia.

Common cases
- Eczema, psoriasis, capillary haemangioma, vitiligo, molluscum contagiosum, Henoch–Schönlein purpura.

Examination of the endocrine system

Examination of the thyroid gland

- Know the signs of hypothyroidism and hyperthyroidism (including eye disease).

Assessment of growth

Assess weight, height, body mass index and puberty (Tanner stages) if allowed. Plot on appropriate growth charts and know how to calculate mid-parental centile. Short stature may be caused by:

- Syndromes associated with abnormal growth, eg Turner's/Noonan syndrome, Russell–Silver syndrome

- Skeletal dysplasia, eg achondroplasia (disproportionate)

- Chronic disease (thin)

- Endocrine disease, eg growth hormone deficiency (increased subcutaneous fat)

- Constitutional delay.

CLINICAL NEURODISABILITY STATION

You have 8 min to perform a specific part of the neurological examination followed by discussion for 5 min. You will be asked to relate your clinical signs to the child's disability. For an older child the standard structured approach should be used.

A pre-school child will not be able to cooperate with a structured examination and the scheme below for examination of the legs should be used. You are unlikely to be asked to examine the cranial nerves or sensation in a young child. A similar approach can be used for the upper limbs. Observing developmental skills, eg jumping or kicking a ball, picking up objects and scribbling, can give useful information about underlying neurological function.

Observation

- Dysmorphic features
- Assess growth, head size and shape; say that you would measure and plot the head circumference, and assess the fontanelle in infants
- Ventricular shunt in the neck
- Look at the child's posture and movements, eg tremor. Is there asymmetry?
- Does the child fix and make eye contact. Is there a squint, nystagmus or ptosis?
- Listen to the child's speech, eg dysarthria. Are there swallowing or bulbar problems?
- Myopathic facies or facial nerve palsy
- Skin lesions of neurocutaneous syndromes
- Look for spectacles, hearing aids, splints, special shoes for clues.

Gait

- Expose legs

- Start by assessing the gait if the child can walk. Types of gait:

  – ataxic gait is broad based and unsteady as a result of a cerebellar problem (normal in toddlers)

  – waddling gait is caused by pelvic girdle weakness, eg muscular dystrophy

  – hemiplegic gait where the leg is extended and circumducted with the foot plantar flexed (toe-walking); the arm may be flexed with hand fisting

  – diplegic gait, which is narrow based and stiff with scissoring

  – high stepping or slapping gait if there is foot drop or peripheral neuropathy

- Gower's sign is positive in proximal weakness (child climbs up his legs from a lying position)

- Is there equal leg length?

- Rheumatological or orthopaedic problems can cause an abnormal gait or limp.

Observation

- Do not examine a child in a wheelchair but transfer him if possible onto a couch

- Examine the back and spine

- Posture, eg frog's leg position in hypotonia, scissoring in diplegia

- Scars from tendon releases

- Fasciculation and wasting, pseudohypertophy in muscular dystrophy.

Tone

- Assess tone by gently lifting and rolling the legs
- Check for normal range of passive movement at the joints, eg ankle plantar flexion, knee extension and hip adduction, and assess for contractures
- Assess for clonus at the ankle
- For the infant, assess tone in the upright and ventral positions, test for head lag and observe sitting.

Power

- This cannot be tested formally in the young child, but watch the child walk and when he moves the legs, or ask the child to 'kick'. Is power normal or reduced?

Coordination

- Test by asking the child to jump (3 years) or hop (5 years)
- Cerebellar signs can be truncal or peripheral. Look for horizontal nystagmus, tremor, past pointing on finger–nose testing.

Reflexes

- Tendon reflexes at the knee and ankle; they can be normal, brisk, reduced or absent (or difficult to illicit?)
- Plantar response is normally down-going after 12 months
- There may be abnormal persistence of the primitive reflexes, eg asymmetrical tonic neck reflex

Signs of an upper motor neuron lesion (UMN)
Increased tone (clasp-knife spasticity), weakness in leg flexors (power may be normal), brisk reflexes, up-going plantars (dorsiflexion of big toe), clonus (four or more beats)

Signs of a lower motor neuron lesion (LMN)
Wasting, reduced tone, power and reflexes

Fasciculation suggests muscle disease

Spinal cord lesion
UMN signs below lesion, LMN signs at the level of the lesion

There may be a sensory level

Common cases
- Hydrocephalus: know the causes of macro- and microcephaly
- Cerebral palsy
- Types: hemiplegia, diplegia, quadriplegia (all with spasticity), ataxic (hypotonia and tremor), dyskinetic (involuntary movements choreoathetosis, dystonia), mixed
- The 'mixed' type of cerebral palsy may have signs of hypotonia and brisk reflexes
- Spinal cord pathology (spina bifida)
- Duchenne muscular dystrophy, myotonic dystrophy
- Neurocutaneous syndromes.

CHILD DEVELOPMENT STATION

This station comprises an 8-min assessment of a child aged less than 4 years followed by a 5-min discussion with the examiner. You will be asked to assess a **specific** aspect of the child's development and then discuss your findings and management. You may also be allowed to take a focused developmental history from the parent, but always confirm this information with assessment. Suitable equipment will be provided and you need to select the most appropriate for the child's developmental age.

You will be asked to assess one of the four areas of development:

1. Gross motor

2. Fine motor and vision

3. Hearing and speech

4. Social and personal.

Learn the age ranges for the key milestones for each area and the age by which most children have attained that skill (limit age).

- Explain to the parent and child what you are doing

- Determine parental concerns if permitted

- Use observation of free play to assess:

  – parent–child interaction

  – child's behaviour, alertness and interest in their surroundings

  – any gross abnormalities, eg dysmorphism or abnormal head shape

- Make the assessment interesting and fun for the child and use praise when appropriate

- Talk to the examiner as you go along

- Start at a level just below the expected age and then work up to the appropriate level, and try to test a skill just beyond the expected age

- Summarise your findings:

the clinical examination

– How confident are you that your assessment is accurate?

– Is the child's development normal or delayed for his or her age?

– Is the delay global or specific?

– What is the nature and severity of the problem?

- Consider what investigations and management are required and which members of the multidisciplinary team should be involved

Below are some key skills and areas to assess in the infant, toddler and pre-school child in the four areas of development.

The infant (eg 9–12 months)

- Gross motor skills: sits well, crawls, stands holding on, forward parachute

- Fine motor and vision: fixes on small object, index finger approach to object and a pincer grasp, looks for fallen toy

- Hearing and speech: responds to name, word with meaning

- Personal and social: waves bye-bye, plays pat-a-cake, may drink from a cup.

The toddler (18 months–2 years)

- Gross motor skills: should walk well, may squat to pick up a toy and kick a ball

- Fine motor and vision: builds a tower of three or four cubes, scribbles and sorts simple shapes

- Hearing and speech: gives object on request, knows or points to two body parts, several words (may join words)

- Personal and social: demonstrates symbolic play, eg brushes doll's hair or feeds.

The pre-school child (3–4 years)

- Gross motor skills: can run and jump, may catch a ball
- Fine motor and vision: makes a train or a bridge from cubes, tripod grasp, copies a circle or cross
- Hearing and speech: can give own name and sex when asked, speaks in short sentences, knows colours
- Personal and social: can remove some clothing, understands taking turns.

Possible cases

- Assess an infant's development
- Assess a 2-year-old child who is not walking
- Assess a 3-year-old child who is not talking.

the clinical examination

INDEX

Note: Questions and answers are indexed by question number. The Clinical Examination section on pages 245–267 is indexed by page number, and the relevant entries are in **bold type**.

PASTEST – DEDICATED TO YOUR SUCCESS

PasTest has been publishing books for medical students and doctors for over 30 years. Our extensive experience means that we are always one step ahead when it comes to knowledge of current trends in Paediatric exams.

We use only the best authors, which enables us to tailor our books to meet your revision needs. We incorporate feedback from candidates to ensure that our books are continually improved.

This commitment to quality ensures that candidates who buy PasTest books achieve successful exam results.

Delivery to your door

With a busy lifestyle, nobody enjoys walking to the shops for something that may or may not be in stock. Let us take the hassle and deliver direct to your door. We will dispatch your book within 24 hours of receiving your order.

How to Order:

www.pastest.co.uk
To order books safely and securely online, shop at our website.

Telephone: +44 (0)1565 752000 Fax: +44 (0)1565 650264
For priority mail order and have your credit card to hand when you call.

Write to us at:
PasTest Ltd
FREEPOST
Haig Road
Parkgate Industrial Estate
Knutsford
WA16 7BR